The Concise Guide to Medical History Taking

Paul Grant

The Concise Guide
to Medical History Taking

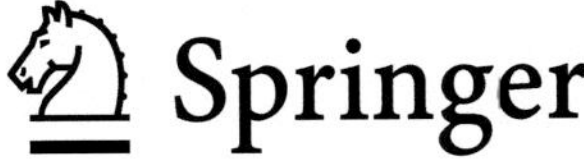 Springer

Paul Grant
Mountfield, UK

ISBN 978-3-031-91473-7   ISBN 978-3-031-91474-4   (eBook)
https://doi.org/10.1007/978-3-031-91474-4

This Springer imprint is published by the registered company Springer Nature Switzerland AG
The registered company address is: Gewerbestrasse 11, 6330 Cham, Switzerland

If disposing of this product, please recycle the paper.

To all my students and those that dedicate themselves to the sheer hard graft of learning medicine.

Foreword

The ability to take a good medical history is a fundamental skill for all healthcare professionals and vital for the delivery of high-quality clinical care. Historically, the patient history gave 90% of the information required to make an accurate clinical diagnosis. Clinical medicine is constantly evolving with medical knowledge expanding daily and new investigations and treatments emerging. However, the ability to take a thorough and accurate history remains a pillar of high-quality clinical care.

Although we now have novel tools and treatments at our disposal, the busy clinical environment presents challenges to the delivery of clinical care. We have an ageing population with an increasing prevalence of chronic disease. Patients attending for assessment may have cognitive decline and require collateral assistance to give a history. We have patients from all parts of the world, who may be giving a history in a second language or with the aid of an interpreter. To overcome these challenges healthcare professionals must be skilled at gathering a history in an organised fashion and able to swiftly identify the key and relevant information required to formulate an accurate differential diagnosis.

With these challenges in mind, Dr Paul Grant, who has extensive experience in the field of medical education and clinical medicine, has produced this excellent textbook, *The Concise Guide to Medical History Taking*. It guides the reader through the process of gathering a medical history and provides a framework to explore a broad range of presenting complaints and medical histories. The book covers the general and sub-specialist areas of clinical medicine and surgery. There is a clear structure to the text, which is intuitive to follow, and the reader is instructed around how to obtain the right information and synthesise the evidence to formulate an accurate diagnosis, which can then be used to direct further investigations and management. There is also guidance on how to summarise findings concisely and present effectively.

The textbook is primarily aimed at student doctors, nurses and physician associates. However, it is also relevant to resident doctors and other more experienced healthcare professionals aiming to deliver high-quality clinical care.

Consultant Physician & Diabetologist   Richard Chudleigh
Singleton Hospital
Associate Professor
Swansea University Medical School
Swansea, UK
November 2024

Competing Interests

The author has no competing interests to declare that are relevant to the content of this manuscript.

Contents

About the Author

Paul Grant is a Consultant Physician and award winning medical educationalist. He is a tutor and dissertation supervisor on the Medical Education MSc course at the University of South Wales. He has previously served as part of the MRCP examinations question writing group and as a PACES examiner. He is the former editor-in-chief of the *British Journal of Diabetes* and *Clinical Medicine* and his previous books include *The Virtual Hospital* (Springer Nature) and *The Gestational Diabetes Survival Guide* (Sheldon Press).

The original version of the book has been revised. A correction to this book can be found at https://doi.org/10.1007/978-3-031-91474-4_15

Chapter 1
Introduction

Abstract Medical history taking is both an art and a logical framework for exploring a wide variety of presenting complaints that healthcare professionals will confront on a daily basis. Taking a good medical history is essential for good patient care.

Traditionally this has been a long and involved process that often lacks focus. The non-specialist may be inexperienced in knowing what key questions are vital.

The approach of this text is to refine the question set for each medical and surgical speciality down to the fundamentals of what meaningful information can be derived, what discriminating details are required and what key things need to be actioned based on the evidence provided.

Keywords Clinical history taking · Differential diagnosis · Red flags · Presenting complaints

A History of Medical History Taking

Anamnesis, derived from the Greek, is the word that refers to the act of remembering or recalling past events, often with a particular focus on memories that have deep, often spiritual or significant meaning [1]. The roots of the word convey the idea of "calling back to mind" or "remembering again". In philosophy, particularly in the works of Plato, *anamnesis* refers to the concept of "recollection".

A medical history reflects the set of information that a Doctor collects through a medical interview. Most medical encounters will involve a history being taken and they vary in their depth and focus depending on the skill and experience of the historian. Data collection is one thing and through careful curation of the content, conclusions, diagnoses and insights can be obtained, leading to the development of a plan of investigations and management.

The practice of taking medical histories has ancient roots and has evolved significantly over centuries, adapting to changes in medical knowledge, cultural beliefs, and diagnostic practices. Hippocrates (c. 460–370 BCE), often called the "Father of Medicine," was among the first to highlight the importance of a systematic approach

P. Grant, *The Concise Guide to Medical History Taking*, https://doi.org/10.1007/978-3-031-91474-4_1

to patient care [2]. During the Islamic Golden Age (eighth–fourteenth centuries), scholars like *Avicenna* (Ibn Sina) and *Rhazes* (Al-Razi) advanced medical history-taking significantly. Avicenna's *Canon of Medicine* focussed on structured patient history taking, distinguishing symptoms of different diseases and encouraging careful observation and questioning [3]. This text influenced European medicine for centuries. By the sixteenth century, doctors like *Paracelsus* and *Andreas Vesalius* flagged direct observation and recording patient details as critical for accurate diagnosis [4]. By the late nineteenth century, the idea of a standardised "case history" emerged. British and American physicians began using written records to document patient histories systematically, including family history, personal habits, and environmental factors [5].

The modern structure of a medical history traditionally consists of identifying the chief presenting complaint and then exploring the specific details of its onset and duration, with questions relevant to the condition focussed at first and then spreading to other relevant areas [6]. This can often require a great deal of speciality specific knowledge and interpretation. Following on from this is enquiring about the patient's past medical history to enable the positioning of the presenting complaint in the context of the individual's previous medical and surgical problems. This then extends to details of the patient's medication given the importance of their current pharmacopoeia. Given the impact of genetics in many illnesses, the next stage is to take a family history, which often indicates potential hereditary risks. More detail is then obtained about the social and environmental aspects of their life, what is their current living situation, ability to function, occupational details, lifestyle issues, alcohol, and smoking habits, which all play a part in the biopsychosocial model of disease. Finally, a general review of body systems has a vital checklist function to assess whether there are other issues which may have been overlooked, both related and unrelated to the presenting problem. This all then leads to the summary—a concise overview of the patient's problems and priorities, the diagnostic hypotheses and the follow up actions that need to be taken to manage the patient safely and effectively.

This structured approach helps ensure that no critical details are missed and provides a clear picture of the patient's overall health status [7].

This book therefore aims to support you, the clinician detective, in extracting the key information required to formulate a diagnosis and an action plan. Each chapter will include the presenting complaints in each system, the questions required to garner a good, relevant medical history, what they mean and the differential diagnoses and suggested investigations that naturally follow on. Red flags i.e. signs of potential malignant disease or critical illness, will also be highlighted.

Objectives
- To provide a clear set of succinct questions for each medical and surgical speciality to train healthcare professionals about what to ask to develop an optimal medical history.

- To ensure that healthcare professionals understand why the questions are being asked in a specific context to help them make a meaningful interpretation of the responses.
- To highlight the red flags / problem areas for each area of medicine to ensure that clinicians are not missing any significant conditions such as malignant disease.

The benefit of this text is that it is aimed at a broad range of healthcare professionals, it is up to date, concise and is based on real world specialist experience from clinical practice and the consultations that take place in a virtual hospital—which is a new approach to information gathering and based on feedback, iteration and suggestions from active clinicians across a wide range of specialities [8].

How to Take a Good Medical History

Some general communication skills which apply to all patient consultations [9] include:

- Active listening—through body language and your verbal and non-verbal responses to what the patient has said.
- An appropriate level of eye contact throughout the consultation.
- Open, relaxed, yet professional body language.
- Don't interrupt. Stop talking and listen to your patient! A key skill commonly overlooked by impatient, inattentive and ill-mannered clinicians.
- Establishing rapport e.g. asking the patient how they are and offering them a seat, being warm and accommodating.
- Demonstrating empathy in response to patient cues: both verbal and non-verbal.
- Summarising at regular intervals, this involves explaining to the patient what you have discussed so far and what you plan to discuss next.

Use open questions to explore the patient's presenting complaint:

- *"What's brought you in to see me today?"*
- *"Tell me about the issues you've been experiencing."*

Provide the patient with enough time to answer and avoid interrupting them.
    Facilitate the patient to expand on their presenting complaint if required:

- *"Ok, can you tell me more about that?"*
- *"Are you able to say a bit more?"*

Traditional Structure of a Medical History [7, 10, 11]

Presenting complaint	Ask the patient to explain and describe as best they can, the nature or character of the specific problem or problems they are experiencing.
	If possible, what is the location of the problem and does it spread, or radiate elsewhere?
	How severe or intense is the problem - how does it impact the patient's ability to function?
History of presenting complaint	The time course of the problem is important to establish. When and how did it start? Does it come and go? How has it progressed?
Triggers	What are the exacerbating and relieving factors?
	What has the patient done to ameliorate the problem?
Associated symptoms	Do they have any other problems allied to the presenting complaint, for example shortness of breath as well as chest pain?
Past medical history	Do you have any medical conditions?
	Have you had any previous operations or procedures?
	Have you ever been hospitalised before?
	Are you currently under the care of a specialist?
	Find out if these pre-existing conditions are under control.
Medications	Do you take any prescribed medications at the moment?
	Can you tell me the names, doses and how often you taken them?
	Do you get any side effects from your medications?
	How often do you forget or don't get round to taking your medications?
	Are you taking any herbal remedies, supplements or over the counter treatments?
Allergies	Are you allergic to anything at all?
	If so, what kind of reaction did you have?
Family history	Is there a history of any medical problems running in your family, for example Diabetes, Heart Disease, Cancer?
	Are both your parents still alive?
	Did they have any medical problems?
	Can you remember what they died from and how old they might have been?
	Do you have any brothers or sisters—are they fit and well?
	Is there anyone in your family who died of a heart condition at a young age?
	Do you know of any unusual illnesses among your relatives?

(continued)

Social history	What are your current living arrangements—where do you live at the moment?
	Who's at home with you?
	What kind of accommodation is it?
	Are you able to get around your home okay?
	Do you have any special adaptations or equipment?
	Are you able to manage with day-to-day tasks by yourself of do you need any help?
	Do you have any home help or carers?
	How often do they visit?
	Are you working at the moment or are you retired?
	What do you do / what did you do for a living?
	Have you ever been exposed to radiation or asbestos?
	How much physical exercise do you do each week?
	Do you have any interesting hobbies or pastimes such as keeping birds?
	Do you have any pets?
	Do you drink much alcohol?
	Quantify the number of units per week.
	If excessive, ask the CAGE screening questions
	Are you a smoker?
	How long have you been addicted to nicotine for?
	Quantify the number of pack years.
	Do you take any recreational drugs such as cannabis or angel dust, PCP etc.?

Systems review (a general screen to check for problems across the whole body)

General	Weight loss, fevers, sweats, fatigue, anorexia
Cardiac	Chest pain, palpitations, leg swelling
Respiratory	Shortness of breath, cough, wheeze, pleurisy
Gastrointestinal	Change in bowel habit, jaundice, abdominal pain, nausea
Neurological	Weakness, sensory disturbances, headache, confusion
Musculoskeletal	Muscle and joint aches and pains, weakness, stiffness
Dermatological	Skin rashes, pruritus, pigmentation, hair or nail changes
Psychological	Mood, well-being, energy levels, memory, concentration

Ideas, Concerns and Expectations

Explore the patient's ideas about the current issue:

- *"What do you think the problem is?"*
- *"What are your thoughts about what is happening?"*
- *"It's clear that you've given this a lot of thought and it would be helpful to hear what you think might be going on."*

Explore the patient's current concerns:

- *"Is there anything, in particular, that's worrying you?"*
- *"What's your number one concern regarding this problem at the moment?"*
- *"What's the worst thing you were thinking it might be?"*

Ask what the patient hopes to gain from the consultation:

- *"What were you hoping I'd be able to do for you today?"*
- *"What would ideally need to happen for you to feel today's consultation was a success?"*
- *"What do you think might be the best plan of action?"*

Closing the Consultation

Summarise the key points back to the patient.

Ask the patient if they have any questions or concerns that have not been addressed.

Thank the patient for their time and let them know what is going to happen next.

Presenting Your History

YOU are the historian, not the patient, so when you come to present to colleagues or a senior clinician, you need to make sure that you present in a clear, organised and professional manner, with considered and intelligent judgements and not bore your audience with waffle and irrelevancies.

Be confident, start with a concise background summary to the patient before launching into the details of the current problem, don't guess or report false information, avoid bias and only highlight pertinent negatives. End with a short summary, restating the most relevant information and your initial impression or differential diagnosis. For example, *"In summary, this is a 50-year-old male with a history of hypertension and type 2 diabetes, presenting with two days of exertional dyspnoea and central crushing chest pain radiating to the left arm. The pain is concerning for potential angina, and further evaluation for acute coronary syndrome is warranted"*.

Despite the expansion of modern diagnostic and imaging tools, there is good evidence that clinicians can still make a diagnosis for most patients using the history on its own [12].

Presenting in this clear, structured way not only ensures important details are covered but also helps the listener quickly grasp the most critical aspects of the patient's health for informed clinical decision-making. Performance will significantly improve with practice (and the use of this book).

References

1. Lombardo F, Pallotti F, Cargnelutti F, Lenzi A. Anamnesis and physical examination. In: Simoni M, Huhtaniemi I, editors. Endocrinology of the testis and male reproduction, Endocrinology. Cham: Springer; 2017.
2. Yapijakis C. Hippocrates of Kos, the father of clinical medicine, and Asclepiades of Bithynia, the father of molecular medicine. Review. In Vivo. 2009;23(4):507–14.
3. Nasser M, Tibi A, Savage-Smith E. Ibn Sina's canon of medicine: 11th century rules for assessing the effects of drugs. J R Soc Med. 2009;102(2):78–80.
4. Zampieri F, ElMaghawry M, Zanatta A, Thiene G. Andreas Vesalius: celebrating 500 years of dissecting nature. Glob Cardiol Sci Pract. 2015;2015(5):66.
5. Sohn AP. 19th-century academic examinations for physicians in the United States Army Medical Department. West J Med. 1994;160(5):472–4.
6. Summerton N. The medical history as a diagnostic technology. Br J Gen Pract. 2008;58(549):273–6.
7. Boston University Medical Campus. Guidelines for the history and physical exam write up. 2008. https://www.google.com/url?sa=t&source=web&rct=j&opi=89978449&url=https://www.bumc.bu.edu/im-residency/files/2010/10/History-and-Physical-Exam-Guidelines.doc&ved=2ahUKEwjgyP_omtqKAxWKVkEAHflROBMQFnoECA8QAQ&usg=AOvVaw07I71yo6enbX_-NMb7msAN. Accessed 23rd June 2024.
8. Grant P. The virtual hospital. Springer; 2024. ISBN: 9783031699436
9. Neighbour R. The inner consultation: how to develop an effective and intuitive consulting style. 2nd ed. Radcliffe; 2005. ISBN: 9781857756791
10. Ball JW, Dains JE, Flynn JA, Solomon BS, Stewart RW. Seidel's guide to physical examination. 9th ed. Mosby; 2018.
11. Tierney LM, Henderson MC, Smetana GW. The patient history: an evidence-based approach to differential diagnosis. 2005.
12. Paley L, Zornitzki T, Cohen J, Friedman J, Kozak N, Schattner A. Utility of clinical examination in the diagnosis of emergency department patients admitted to the department of medicine of an academic hospital. Arch Intern Med. 2011;171(15):1394–6. https://doi.org/10.1001/archinternmed.2011.340. PMID: 21824956

Chapter 2
The Cardiac System

Abstract The cardiac system is a vital component of the human organism and failures of both the pump and circulatory elements are significant contributors to illness. Cardiovascular disease, exacerbated by western lifestyles, is the leading cause of death in developed countries. Understanding how symptoms are manifested from the underlying pathophysiology is important in identifying the diagnosis. Carefully exploring signs and symptoms is a key skill as many patients, even those with marked heart disease may present with minimal clues.

One of the commonest presenting complaints to emergency departments and the acute medical unit is chest pain, and once declared 'troponin-negative, non-cardiac' the search is often given up. This is the wrong approach, and we must endeavour to discover what ails our patients even if it doesn't fit into a neat box.

Keywords Angina · Congestive cardiac failure · Arrhythmias · Myocardial infarction · Pericarditis · Aortic dissection

Introduction

Cardiology is an important medical speciality because compromises of the cardiovascular system can have important implications for health and wellbeing [1]. The manifestations of cardiac disturbance need to be taken seriously and evaluated promptly. This is especially relevant given its impact on the high levels of morbidity and mortality in the western world [2]. In this chapter we will explore the common cardiac presenting complaints and differential diagnoses, which are summarised in Table 2.1, the common cardiac conditions that present in day to day clinical practice along with their commonly associated constellation of symptoms (Table 2.2), followed by the essential details that need to be gathered regarding the patient's background. The main bulk of the chapter then breaks down each common presenting complaints and indicates the key questions, based on expert opinion, that need to be asked along with their rationale and the approach to management [3–5].

P. Grant, *The Concise Guide to Medical History Taking*,
https://doi.org/10.1007/978-3-031-91474-4_2

Table 2.1 Common cardiac presenting complaints [3]

Cardiac system presenting complaints	Commonly associated conditions
Chest pain	Acute coronary syndrome (ACS, from angina to myocardial infarction)
	Pericarditis
	Aortic dissection
	Pulmonary embolism
	Pneumonia / pleurisy
	Pneumothorax
	Gastro-oesphageal reflux
	Oesophageal spasm
	Musculo-skeletal pain
	Costochondritis
	Stress / anxiety
Shortness of breath / dyspnoea	Cardiac failure
	Coronary artery disease / angina
	Arrhythmias
	Asthma
	COPD
	Pneumonia / pleurisy
	Pulmonary embolism
	Pneumothorax
	Interstitial lung disease
	Pleural effusion
	Anaemia
	Carbon monoxide poisoning
	Acidosis
	Sepsis
	Stress / anxiety
Palpitations	Arrhythmias
	Heart disease
	Valve disorders
	Stress / anxiety
	Stimulants e.g. caffeine, alcohol, nicotine, narcotics, medications
	Hyperthyroidism
	Menopause
	Systemic disease e.g. anaemia, pyrexia, dehydration

(continued)

Table 2.1 (continued)

Cardiac system presenting complaints	Commonly associated conditions
Syncope	Arrythmias
	Structural heart disease e.g. valve disorders or cardiomyopathy
	Heart block
	Vaso-vagal syncope
	Postural hypotension
	Autonomic dysfunction
	Situational syncope
	Seizures
	Cerebrovascular disease
	Hypoglycaemia
	Medications e.g. anti-hypertensives, beta blockers
Oedema	Heart failure
	Chronic venous insufficiency, deep vein thrombosis
	Renal disease
	Liver disease
	Lymphoedema
	Medications e.g. calcium channel blockers, NSAID's, steroids, hormonal contraceptives (OCP)
	Hypothyroidism
	Cushing's syndrome
	Infections and inflammatory conditions
	Pregnancy

Background History for the Cardiac System

Several medical conditions affecting the cardiac system can run in families and a large number of genetic, dietary and environmental factors can play a part, so before you get into too much detail about the presenting problems it's useful to establish the following [3, 5, 7].

- History of previous medical or surgical problems affecting the cardiac or respiratory system and any previous investigations such as echocardiography or angiography?
- Associated conditions e.g. diabetes, high cholesterol, other chronic diseases?
- Do they have a family history of any cardiac or cholesterol related conditions, (especially ischaemic heart disease at a young age as this may suggest a genetic component)?
- Medications—multiple drugs, both prescribed and recreational, can impact the heart. Make sure that you get a full list of what they are taking and why. Any recently stopped or started medications?

Table 2.2 Common cardiac conditions and associated signs and symptoms [2, 6]

Common cardiac conditions	Common symptoms
Angina	Caused by reduced blood flow to the heart, often due to coronary artery disease. It typically presents as pressure or tightness in the chest.
Aortic dissection	A tear in the inner layer of the aorta, leading to severe, tearing chest pain that can radiate to the back.
Arrhythmias	Irregular heartbeats, such as atrial fibrillation, supraventricular tachycardia, or premature ventricular contractions, can cause palpitations and breathlessness.
Cardiac failure	When the heart can't pump blood effectively, fluid can build up in the lungs, causing dyspnoea, particularly when lying down (orthopnoea) as well as oedema, fatigue and chest pain.
Heart block	A delay or blockage in the heart's electrical system may be asymptomatic or can cause bradycardia (slow heart rate) and result in light headedness, fatigue, syncope, dyspnoea and occasional palpitations.
Myocardial Infarction	A more severe form of angina where blood flow to part of the heart is blocked, leading to damage of the heart muscle. Can present with severe, central, 'crushing' chest, arm and jaw pain, dyspnoea and distress.
Pericarditis	Inflammation of the pericardium, the sac surrounding the heart, often causing sharp, stabbing pain that may worsen with deep breathing or lying down. Often relieved by sitting forwards.
Valve disorders	Heart valve disorders occur when one or more of the heart's valves do not function properly, either by not opening fully (stenosis) or not closing properly (regurgitation or insufficiency). These issues can affect the flow of blood through the heart and the body, leading to fatigue, dyspnoea, palpitations, chest pain and peripheral oedema. Neurological symptoms may include light headedness and syncope.

- Constitutional upset—have you lost any weight recently? Has your diet or eating patterns changed? Is it more difficult to undertake your regular activities? Any major life events recently?
- Alcohol and smoking history—this is very relevant to cardiac conditions. Do you use any recreational drugs? Caffeine intake?

CHEST PAIN = discomfort in the chest, classically the front [5, 8]

Onset + Duration
- When did it start / how long has it been going on for?

Acute, sudden pain is more likely to be due to an ACS or PE.
Prolonged pain can be associated with aortic dissection, GORD or MSK pain.

Character
- How best would you describe your chest pain?
- Is it dull / sharp / tight?

The character provides clues to the underlying aetiology. Sharp or tight pains are less likely to be cardiac. Aortic dissection is typically described as excruciating, tearing, or ripping pain.

Severity
- How severe has your chest pain been at its worst?
- 1 means the slightest discomfort and 10 means the worst pain imaginable.

Intense pain could indicate a large area of the heart is affected, but milder pain does not rule out ACS.

Location
- Whereabouts are you experiencing the chest pain?

Chest pain can originate from various structures, including the heart, lungs, oesophagus, muscles, bones, and nerves. By assessing the location, clinicians can narrow down the possible causes.

Radiation
- Does the pain spread anywhere?

ACS pain may radiate upwards to the neck, jaw, or even the teeth. This type of pain is often referred pain and may not be immediately recognised as cardiac in origin. Pain from acid reflux or a hiatal hernia can be felt in the lower chest or upper abdomen and may be associated with eating or lying down.

Provocation
- Did anything trigger the pain?
- What were you doing at the time?

Exertion or physical activity is more likely to indicate an ACS.
Pain on rest could suggest unstable angina.
Postural factors implicate MSK pain or pericarditis.
Breathing or coughing suggests pleurisy or a pneumothorax.
Eating and drinking is associated with GORD or oesophageal spasm.

Relief
- Is there anything that helps to relieve the pain?

Resting, leaning forward, lying down, taking a GTN spray may all help reduce the chest pain. Pain that lessens with rest can be associated with both ACS and MSK pain.

Leaning forward is classic for pericarditis. Antacids help with GORD.

Holding breath or breathing slowly can improve pleuritic pain.

Associations
- Do you get any other symptoms at the same time as the chest pain?
- E.g. palpitations, shortness of breath, nausea, dizziness.

Nausea and vomiting, sweating, dyspnoea and disorientation are all common with an ACS.

Dyspnoea can be due to cardiac failure or PE.

Upper GI symptoms can occur with GORD.

Common Causes of Chest Pain [9]

Cardiac	Acute coronary syndrome, aortic dissection, pericarditis.
Respiratory	Pneumonia, pulmonary emboli, pneumothorax.
Gastro-intestinal	Hiatus hernia, gastro-oesophageal reflux disease, peptic ulcer disease.
MSK	Musculo-skeletal chest pain (trauma or exertion), costochondritis.
Psychological	Stress, anxiety, panic.

Approach to Management

Central and peripheral cardiovascular examination is important. Don't forget to listen to the lung bases and listen carefully for cardiac murmurs. Musculo-skeletal pain is often reproducible on palpation but be gentle [10].

Check basic observations including blood pressure, pulse and oxygen saturations.

Blood tests	FBC, U&E's, LFT's, Clotting studies, Troponin (on admission and at 8–12 h).
Imaging	Chest X-Ray (for all), CT chest if dissection suspected (urgent). CTPA for PE.
Other	ECG.
	Echocardiography.
	ABG and Well's score if VTE suspected.
	Upper GI endoscopy (if GORD suspected) plus H. Pylori serology.
Treatment	Analgesia, trial of nitrates, oxygen. Treat the underlying cause.
Red flags	Sudden onset severe chest pain (potential MI or dissection).
	Shortness of breath and abnormal ECG—right heart strain (possible PE).
	Radiating pain 'tearing / ripping' (possible dissection).
	Haemodynamic instability (cardiogenic shock).

SHORTNESS OF BREATH (SOB) / DYSPNOEA = the uncomfortable feeling of having difficulty breathing [11]

Character
- Can you describe what it's like for you to breath at the moment?
- Is it tightness, heaviness, or an inability to get enough air?

Different people mean different things by shortness of breath, it's best to capture verbatim what they mean 'difficulty breathing' is different to 'rapid breathing' or 'having a tight chest'.

Onset + Duration
- When did it start / how long has it been going on for?
- Was it sudden or gradually progressive?
- Does it come and go?

Sudden onset SOB is more likely to be associated with acute coronary syndromes, pulmonary emboli, pneumothoraces or acute exacerbations of underlying lung diseases.
Progressive SOB may be linked to cardiac failure, infectious respiratory disease or underlying insidious conditions such as anaemia.

Severity
- How severe is the shortness of breath on a scale of 1–10?
Patients can give a good gauge as to the severity of their breathlessness and this is commonly linked to the severity of the underlying respiratory compromise.

Triggers and Relieving Factors
- Is it worse at certain times of day, like at night or early morning?
- Is there anything that makes it better or worse?

Are there any obvious situational, environmental or postural precipitants?

Associations
- Do you have a cough?
- If so, is it productive, what colour is the sputum, any blood?
- Have you had any wheezing?
- Any bluish discolouration of your lips or fingers?

Airway irritation and infections can often lead to a cough, if sputum is being produced make sure that you take a look and note its characteristics.
Wheeze suggests a restrictive lung disease or pulmonary oedema (cardiac wheeze).
Blue discolouration is a feature of central and peripheral cyanosis.

Common Causes of Shortness of Breath [12]

Cardiac	Acute coronary syndromes, cardiac failure, arrhythmias, valve disease.
Respiratory	Pneumonia, pulmonary emboli, pneumothorax, asthma, COPD, pleural effusion, upper airway obstruction.
MSK	Musculo-skeletal chest pain, trauma.
Psychological	Stress, anxiety, panic.
Metabolic	Anaemia, acidosis, obesity, pregnancy.

Approach to Management

Dyspnoea is a common symptom with causes ranging from benign conditions like anxiety, to life-threatening ones such as PE. Identifying the underlying system involved is crucial for accurate diagnosis and management [13, 14]. Cardiovascular examination is useful to assess whether there is an obvious cause of lung or heart compromise. Don't forget to examine the periphery for signs of systemic illness and oedema. Start with an ABC assessment.

Blood tests	FBC, U&E's, inflammatory markers if infection suspected.
Imaging	Chest X-Ray, CTPA if PE suspected.
Other	ECG.
	Arterial blood gas.
	Well's score if VTE suspected. Consider D-Dimers.
	Peak flow / lung function tests.
Treatment	Reassurance, sit upright, oxygen if hypoxic, inhalers / nebulisers if wheeze (in the context of known underlying lung disease)
	Antibiotics if suspected lower respiratory infection.
	Treat the underlying cause.
	ITU review if failure to respond / deterioration in ventilation.
Red flags	Haemoptysis, hypoxia, abnormal ECG (don't forget the signs of right heart strain i.e. RVH, S1, Q3, T3 etc.)

PALPITATIONS = the sensation of having a racing or erratic heart beat [15, 16]

Character
- Can you describe what you mean by palpitations?
- Are you able to tap out the rhythm?
- Do you feel as if your heart is beating too fast or too slow?

Palpitations could consist of fluttering, pounding, racing, skipping beats or an irregularity of the heartbeat.

Onset + Duration
- When did it start / how long has it been going on for?
- Have things been worsening over time?

Clarify the time course of the development of the palpitations. Was it sudden onset or gradual and does it come and go?

Frequency
- How often do you get the palpitations?
  Ascertain whether they occur daily, weekly, or just intermittently?

Severity
- On a scale of 1 to 10, how would you rate the intensity of the palpitations?

Triggers and Relieving Factors
- Have you noticed anything that brings it on?
- Is there anything that makes it better or worse?

Is there an identifiable precipitant—during exercise / rest / lying down / stress / coffee / specific situations?

Associations
- Do you experience any chest pains?
- Do you get short of breath?
- Do you feel lightheaded, dizzy or you might faint?
- Do you sweat excessively?
- How would you describe your stress levels recently?

Palpitations could be linked to ischaemic heart disease.
Dyspnoea suggests both cardiac and respiratory involvement.
Dizziness and sweating suggest cardiovascular insufficiency.
Recent stress could suggest anxiety or an underlying endocrine disorder. Look for a correlation with stressful life events.

Common Causes of Palpitations [17]

Cardiac	Arrhythmias e.g. Atrial fibrillation, Atrial flutter. Valve disease e.g. mitral valve prolapse. Structural heart disease e.g. hypertrophic cardiomyopathy, cardiac failure.
Respiratory	COPD, Pulmonary emboli.
Endocrine	Hyperthyroidism, Hypoglycaemia, Phaeochromocytoma (rare but not to be missed).
Haematologic	Anaemia—can lead to tachycardia and palpitations as the body tries to compensate.
Psychological	Anxiety and panic disorders, depression.
Stimulants	Caffeine, nicotine, cocaine, amphetamines, beta-agonists, levothyroxine. Additionally, withdrawal from alcohol, benzodiazepines, or other substances can lead to palpitations.
Metabolic	Hypo and hyperkalaemia, hypo and hypercalcaemia affect the cardiac action potential and can lead to arrhythmias and the manifestation of palpitations.
Neurological	Vaso-vagal syncope, postural orthopaedic tachycardia syndrome (POTS).

Approach to Management

Understanding the potential causes of palpitations across these body systems can help guide further investigation and management [18]. Assess for features of haemodynamic compromise. Refer to a Cardiology specialist.

Blood tests	FBC, U&E's, Calcium, Magnesium, TFT's, Inflammatory markers, blood glucose, Troponin.
	Catecholamines / metanephrines if Phaeochromocytoma suspected.
	Drug screening / toxicology.
Imaging	CXR, Echocardiography, Cardiac MRI (after discussion with Cardiology)
Other	ECG
	Exercise ECG
	Ambulatory ECG e.g. Holter monitor, event recorder, implantable loop recorder
	Electrophysiological studies.
	Tilt table test.
	Psychiatric assessment.
	Symptom diary.
Treatment	Reassurance, cardiac monitoring, remove any precipitants.
	Correct any underlying medical conditions.
	Mindfulness and relaxation techniques where appropriate.
Red flags	Associated chest pain could suggest ACS [19].
	Signs of cardiac failure.
	Syncope or pre-syncope could indicate a serious arrhythmia.
	Family history of sudden cardiac death at a young age.

SYNCOPE = fast onset, short duration loss of consciousness [20]

Character
- How would you describe the sensation?

Individuals may use a variety of terms from dizziness to fainting to describe their experience.

Onset + Duration
- When did it start?
- Was it sudden or gradual?
- What were you doing at the time?
- How long did it last for?
- Has this happened before?

What was the patient doing just before e.g. sitting, standing, exercising.

Prodrome
- Did you get any warning signs before it started?
- Flashing lights, headaches, chest pains, change in vision?

Establish any features of neurological or cardiac involvement.

Recovery
- How long did it take before you felt back to normal?
- Did you feel confused or disorientated afterwards?

Establish whether this was a transient episode that led to a quick resolution like a vaso-vagal, or a more complex phenomenon.

Eyewitness
- Was there a witness?
- How would they describe what happened?
- Were there any features of a seizure? E.g. tongue-biting, incontinence.

Witness reports can be very useful in providing more detail as the patient themselves may not have realised everything that was happening at the time.

Associations
- Did you feel your heart racing or skipping beats before the loss of consciousness?
- Did you experience any chest pain or shortness of breath?
- Did you have a headache or feel nauseated?
- Any visual changes such as loss of vision, field changes or double vision?

Look for features of cardiac compromise or neurological issues.

Common Causes of Cardiac Syncope [21]

Cardiac	Arrhythmias e.g. AV block, VT, VF, SVT, long QT syndrome
	Structural heart disease; Aortic stenosis, Mitral valve prolapse, Hypertrophic cardiomyopathy, pulmonary hypertension.
	Ischaemic heart disease.
	Cardiac tamponade.
	Acute decompensated cardiac failure.

Approach to Management

Identifying the specific cause of cardiac syncope is crucial, as some causes are life-threatening and require urgent intervention [22]. This section focuses on the cardiac work up and there is more detail in the neurology section. Physical examination needs to evaluate cardiovascular signs, such as heart murmurs, blood pressure, and pulse abnormalities.

Blood tests	FBC, U&E's, Calcium, Magnesium, Troponin.
Imaging	CXR, Echocardiography
Other	ECG
	Ambulatory ECG monitoring
	Stress testing
	Tilt table testing
	Electrophysiological studies
Treatment	Symptom / events diary
	Manage the underlying cause
	Emergency calls button or remote monitors (especially for those who live alone).
Red flags	Syncope that occurs during physical activity, particularly in young individuals, suggests serious underlying causes like hypertrophic cardiomyopathy, aortic stenosis, or arrhythmias.
	Sudden syncope without any prodromal symptoms (such as dizziness or nausea) can indicate an arrhythmic cause, like ventricular tachycardia or complete heart block.
	Family history of sudden cardiac death.
	Patients with implanted devices (pacemaker or a defibrillator) who experience syncope may be experiencing device malfunction or progression of their underlying heart disease.

OEDEMA = fluid retention in the body's tissues [23]

Location
- Whereabouts are you getting the tissue swelling?
- Is it more pronounced in one area or is it generalised?
- Was there any trauma or injuries to that area?

Distribution and symmetry of the oedema is important e.g. hands, feet, ankles, legs, face, abdomen (anasarca). Ask about recent injuries / knocks and bumps.

Onset + Duration
- When did the swelling start / how long has it been going on for?
- Does the swelling come and go?
- Did it develop gradually or suddenly?

Time course and changes in oedema are useful to understand in relation to potential underlying causes.

Progression
- Has the swelling been getting worse over time or staying the same?
- Are there any patterns e.g. worse at the end of the day, does it get worse with elevation?
- What makes the swelling better or worse?

The patient may provide clues as to anything that makes the oedema better or worse—positional factors, activity, heat.

Immobility
- Have you had any recent long periods of immobility? (e.g., long flights, bed rest).
- What is your occupation?

Oedema can develop due to prolonged immobilisation.

Associations
- Do you experience any chest pain or shortness of breath?
- Do you have any cough, wheezing, or fatigue?

May suggest cardiac failure and pulmonary oedema.

- Do you experience any abdominal discomfort, bloating, or weight gain?

May suggest greater levels of oedema if abdominal involvement.

- Is there any pain or tenderness associated with the swelling?
- Do you have any history of varicose veins or blood clots?

Could indicate vascular involvement or thrombosis (especially if unilateral).

- Are you pregnant or have you recently been pregnant? (Ask all young women).
- Any history of thyroid disease?
- Fatigue, cold intolerance, weight gain?

Hypothyroidism can lead to peripheral oedema and cardiac failure.

- Any background history of liver disease?

Ask about jaundice, pruritus and dark urine.

Common Causes of Oedema [24]

Cardiac	Congestive cardiac failure, valve disease, cardiomyopathy
Respiratory	Chronic lung disease
Vascular	Thrombophlebitis, varicose veins, deep vein thrombosis.
Metabolic	Hypoalbuminaemia, malnutrition, hypothyroidism, pregnancy, renal impairment
Medication	Oral contraceptive pill, calcium channel blockers, NSAIS's, steroids.

Approach to Management

Oedema can be a symptom of an underlying health condition, particularly if it is persistent, or there are other significant symptoms (such as dyspnoea) [25]. General examination is useful to evaluate other body systems. Map the extent and distribution of the oedema, note whether it is pitting in nature or not, and the colour of the overlying skin. Ensure that you look for other features of congestive cardiac failure.

Blood tests	FBC, U&E's, LFT's, Albumin, urine protein, BNP, TFT's, HbA1c, HCG.
Imaging	CXR, lower limb ultrasound / doppler evaluation, Echocardiography.
Treatment	General measures include encouraging mobilisation and elevation of the legs when at rest. Compression stockings if no contraindications may be helpful. Avoid standing for long periods of time.
	Treat the underlying cause.
	Caution with diuretics in the context of renal impairment.
Red flags	Associated abdominal wall oedema.
	Decompensated congestive cardiac failure.
	Unilateral hot swollen hard lower limb—need to rule out VTE.

INTERESTING FACT: The most heart attacks happen on Christmas Day, followed by Boxing Day and New Year's Day [26]. However, more heart attacks occur on a Monday than any other day of the week.

References

1. NHS England, GIRFT. Cardiology. 2024. https://gettingitrightfirsttime.co.uk/medical_specialties/cardiology/. Accessed 12 Feb 2024.
2. World Health Organisation. Cardiovascular diseases. 2021. https://www.who.int/news-room/fact-sheets/detail/cardiovascular-diseases-(cvds). Accessed 12 Feb 2024.
3. Peart P. Cardiovascular history taking and clinical examination. Clin Integr Care. 2022;12:100105. ISSN 2666-8696
4. Narasimman A, Choudhari SG. Redefining clinical skills in history taking in association with epidemiological assessment of risk factors, and diagnosis of patients with cardiovascular diseases with a special emphasis on COVID-19. Cureus. 2022;14(10):e30829.
5. National Institute for Health and Care Excellence. Clinical knowledge summary. What history should I take from a person with chest pain? 2022. https://cks.nice.org.uk/topics/chest-pain/diagnosis/history/. Accessed 24 Feb 2024.
6. Heart Research Institute. The 12 most common heart and cardiovascular conditions and what you can do about them. 2024. https://www.hriuk.org/health/learn/cardiovascular-disease/the-12-most-common-heart-and-cardiovascular-conditions-and-what-you-can-do-about-them. Accessed 24 Feb 2024.
7. Boston University Medical Campus. Guidelines for the history and physical exam write up. 2008. https://www.google.com/url?sa=t&source=web&rct=j&opi=89978449&url=https://www.bumc.bu.edu/im-residency/files/2010/10/History-and-Physical-Exam-Guidelines.doc&ved=2ahUKEwjgyP_omtqKAxWKVkEAHflROBMQFnoECA8QAQ&usg=AOvVaw07I71yo6enbX_-NMb7msAN. Accessed 23 June 2024.
8. BMJ Best Practice. Assessment of chest pain. London: BMJ Publishing; 2020a.
9. Bösner S, Becker A, Haasenritter J, et al. Chest pain in primary care: epidemiology and pre-work-up probabilities. Eur J Gen Pract. 2009;15(3):141–6.
10. McConaghy JR. Outpatient diagnosis of acute chest pain in adults. Am Fam Physician. 2013;87(3):177–82.
11. National Institute for Health and Care Excellence. Clinical knowledge summary. Breathlessness: how should I assess a person with breathlessness? 2024. https://cks.nice.org.uk/topics/breathlessness/diagnosis/assessment/. Accessed 25 Feb 2024.
12. BMJ Best Practice. Assessment of dyspnoea. BMJ Publishing; 2022. https://bestpractice.bmj.com. Accessed 25 Feb 2024.
13. Coggle S, Jolly E, Firth JD. Acute medical presentations. In: Firth J, Conlon C, Cox T, editors. Oxford textbook of medicine. 6th ed. Oxford: Oxford University Press; 2020.
14. Simon C, Everitt H, van Dorp F, et al. Respiratory medicine. In: Oxford handbook of general practice. 6th ed. Oxford: Oxford University Press; 2020.
15. National Institute for Health and Care Excellence. Clinical knowledge summary. Palpitations: how should I assess a person with palpitations? 2020. https://cks.nice.org.uk/topics/palpitations/diagnosis/assessment/. Accessed 25 Feb 2024.
16. Abbott A. Diagnostic approach to palpitations. Am Fam Physician. 2005;71(4):743–50.
17. BMJ Best Practice. Evaluation of palpitations. BMJ Publishing; 2018. http://bestpractice.bmj.com. Accessed 25 Feb 2024.
18. Fay M, Wolff A. Guidance on the management of palpitations in primary care. Guidelines.co.uk; 2018. http://www.guidelines.co.uk. Accessed 25 Feb 2024.
19. Abi Khalil C, Haddad F, Al Suwaidi J. Investigating palpitations: the role of Holter monitoring and loop recorders. BMJ. 2017;358
20. National Institute for Health and Care Excellence. Clinical Knowledge Summary. How should I assess a person presenting with a blackout or syncope? 2023. https://cks.nice.org.uk/topics/blackouts-syncope/diagnosis/assessment/. Accessed 25 Feb 2024.
21. Brignole M, Moya A, de Lange F, et al. ESC guidelines for the diagnosis and management of syncope. Eur Heart J. 2018a;39(21):1883–948.

22. Sutton R, Ricci F, Fedorowski A. Risk stratification of syncope: current syncope guidelines and beyond. Auton Neurosci. 2021;238
23. National Institute for Health and Care Excellence. Clinical knowledge summary. Heart failure – chronic: what else could it be? 2024. https://cks.nice.org.uk/topics/heart-failure-chronic/diagnosis/what-else-could-it-be/. Accessed 24 Sept 2024.
24. BMJ Best Practice. Assessment of peripheral oedema. BMJ Publishing Group; 2024. http://bestpractice.bmj.com. Accessed 25 Feb 2024.
25. Hayhoe B, Kim D, Aylin PP, et al. Adherence to guidelines in management of symptoms suggestive of heart failure in primary care. Heart. 2019;105(9):678–85.
26. Phillips DP, Jarvinen JR, Abramson IS, Phillips RR. Cardiac mortality is higher around Christmas and New Year's than at any other time: the holidays as a risk factor for death. Circulation. 2004;110(25):3781–8.

Chapter 3
The Respiratory System

Abstract There are two very important structures within the chest. The right lung, and the left lung. They are the foundational organs of the respiratory system, whose most basic function is to facilitate gas exchange from the environment into the bloodstream. In addition, the upper airways, larynx, pharynx and diaphragm all have an important part to play. Understanding how chest related symptoms manifest is crucial as this can provide helpful clues to underlying causes. The lungs only have a limited repertoire of ways to express pathology and dysfunction, namely dyspnoea, cough, wheeze and pleurisy. It is key therefore to use the history of respiratory dysfunction to establish the diagnosis of various disease states and consider whether this is due to pulmonary or extra-pulmonary disease (or both). The lungs are a primary location for a large proportion of human disease. Airways damage can be further classified into obstructive and restrictive deficits so don't forget your spirometry interpretation and the relationships between FEV1 (forced expiratory volume) and FVC (fixed vital capacity).

Keywords Respiratory disease · Pulmonary system · Pleurisy · Pneumonia · Dyspnoea · Cough · Wheeze · Haemoptysis · Sputum · Lungs

Introduction

Respiratory medicine is not just about telling people off for cigarette smoking, it is an advanced medical speciality that aims to overcome serious pathology, improve respiratory function and oxygenation. Respiratory illnesses are incredibly common, and clinicians need to be able to diagnose a wide range of conditions across the whole upper and lower respiratory system which includes the nose, throat, larynx, bronchus, bronchi, lungs and the diaphragm [1]. Table 3.1 provides a summary of the most frequent presenting complaints relating to the respiratory system along with commonly associated differential diagnoses and Table 3.2 lists the commonest pathologies and how they can manifest.

© The Author(s), under exclusive license to Springer Nature Switzerland AG 2025

P. Grant, *The Concise Guide to Medical History Taking*, https://doi.org/10.1007/978-3-031-91474-4_3

Table 3.1 Summary table of respiratory presenting complaints and differential diagnoses [2]

Respiratory system presenting complaints	Commonly associated conditions
Dyspnoea (shortness of breath)	Asthma COPD Pneumonia/pleurisy Pulmonary embolism Pneumothorax Pulmonary fibrosis / Interstitial lung disease (ILD) Pleural effusion
	Cardiac failure Coronary artery disease/angina Arrhythmias
	Anaemia Carbon monoxide poisoning Acidosis (acid / base imbalance) Sepsis
	Stress / anxiety
Cough	Upper respiratory tract infections Lower respiratory tract infections Asthma COPD Lung cancer Pulmonary fibrosis Pulmonary embolism
	Congestive cardiac failure
	Gastro-oesophageal reflux disease Aspiration
	Irritants / pollutants / chemicals / allergens Medications e.g. ACE inhibitors
Haemoptysis	Bronchitis Bronchiectasis Lung cancer Pneumonia Tuberculosis Pulmonary embolism COPD Pulmonary abscess
	Mitral stenosis Congestive cardiac failure Arterio-venous malformations
	Parasitic infections Aspergillosis
	Coagulopathies Anticoagulants e.g. Warfarin
	Goodpasture's syndrome Wegener's granulomatosis

(continued)

Table 3.1 (continued)

Respiratory system presenting complaints	Commonly associated conditions
Wheeze	Asthma COPD Bronchitis Respiratory infections Pulmonary fibrosis Pulmonary oedema Foreign body aspiration Allergic reactions (anaphylaxis)
	Congestive cardiac failure
	Gastro-oesophageal reflux disease Aspiration pneumonitis
Pleurisy/pleuritic chest pain	Pneumonia Pulmonary embolism Pneumonthorax Infections e.g. respiratory viruses, tuberculosis Lung cancer
	Pericarditis Myocardial infarction
	Costochondritis Chest wall trauma
	Systemic Lupus Erythematosus (SLE) Rheumatoid arthritis Scleroderma
Stridor (uncommon)	Foreign body obstruction Vocal fold paralysis
	Larygospasm Pharyngeal wall oedema (anaphylaxis) Space occupying lesion Whooping cough Acute epiglottitis
	Goitre Lymphadenopathy

Table 3.2 Summary table of common respiratory conditions and associated symptoms [3]

Common respiratory conditions	Common symptoms
Asthma	The hallmark of asthma is shortness of breath, cough and wheeze. May be associated with other atopic conditions such as hayfever and eczema and urticaria.
Bronchitis	Inflammation of the bronchial tubes. May be acute or chronic depending on the duration and frequency of symptoms. Presents with dyspnoea, cough with sputum production, chest discomfort, wheeze, raised temperatures and coryzal symptoms.
Bronchiectasis	Chronic scarring of the airways. Presents with recurrent or chronic respiratory infections, chronic productive cough and difficulty in breathing, plus fatigue.
COPD	Long-term, progressive lung disease that causes breathing difficulties. Shortness of breath, chronic cough, increased sputum production, wheezing, chest tightness, fatigue, recurrent infections, sudden symptomatic deteriorations.
Lung cancer	Commonly caused by tobacco smoking. Lung cancers may be asymptomatic until advanced. Can present with chest pain, persistent cough, haemoptysis, dyspnoea, constitutional upset, fatigue and weight loss. Recurrent chest infections or a paraneoplastic syndrome (e.g. SIADH or hypercalcaemia) may be the first sign of underlying disease.
Pneumonia	Fatigue, fever, dyspnoea, pleuritic chest pain, anorexia, weight loss, productive cough.
Pulmonary embolism	Sudden onset dyspnoea, pleuritic chest pain, cough, haemoptysis, haemodyamic instability, abnormal ECG, hypoxia.
Pulmonary fibrosis	Progressive dyspnoea, especially on physical exertion, fatigue, chronic dry cough, weight loss, chest discomfort, clubbing. Poor exercise tolerance. Abnormal lung sounds, wheeze / crackles.
Respiratory tract infections	These can be upper or lower respiratory tract; location affects the predominance of symptoms. Dyspnoea, cough, sputum production, fevers, fatigue, myalgia, anorexia, weight loss, chest pain, coryzal symptoms.
Tuberculosis	Symptoms depend on whether the TB infection is active or latent. Chronic cough, fevers, night sweats, weight loss, fatigue, generalised weakness, chest discomfort, dyspnoea. Lymphadenopathy. Look for extra-pulmonary manifestations.

Background History for the Respiratory System

Many conditions affecting the respiratory system are affected by environmental factors, allergens, occupational exposure and recreational activities such as smoking (not just cigarettes) [1]. Several medical conditions affecting the respiratory system can cause systemic illness and it is important to be comprehensive [4]. Long standing respiratory diseases such as asthma can settle and flare. It's very useful to establish their current treatment course, response to different medications and self-monitoring e.g. peak expiratory flow rates changes over time.

- History of previous medical or surgical problems affecting the lung and any previous investigations such as pulmonary function tests / spirometry, bronchoscopies or operations (lung or otherwise) and immobility?
- How well controlled is any pre-existing disease such as Asthma?
- Do they have a family history of any respiratory conditions in first degree relatives (parents or siblings), noting the age that the disease developed and any causes of death (relevant for conditions such as Cystic Fibrosis for example which is inherited in an autosomal dominant manner).
- Medications—multiple drugs, both prescribed and recreational, can impact the respiratory system. Make sure that you get a full list of what they are taking and what they have tried previously. How often are they are having to use their inhalers or nebulisers?
- Allergies and types of reactions.
- Smoking—when did they start, how much do they smoke? 1 pack = 20 cigarettes. Pack years = years smoked x average number of packs smoked per day.
- General social context—who the patient lives with, ability to perform activities of daily living, need for carers, type of accommodation, local environment (e.g. busy main road, next door to a nuclear power station), close contacts with people who have been travelling abroad. Current and previous occupations (?exposures). Pets and hobbies. Exercise tolerance.
- Explore recent travel history if relevant (location, duration of stay, activities, unwell contacts).
- Constitutional upset—weight loss can suggest malignancy or end stage COPD. Fevers / sweats indicate infection. Night sweats suggest TB. Fatigue can be due to anaemia or malignancy.

SHORTNESS OF BREATH / DYSPNOEA = difficulty in breathing [5]

Character
- What do you mean by shortness of breath?

For different people this could be difficulty catching their breath, breathing very rapidly or pain on breathing. Try to clarify what they actually mean.

Onset + Duration
- When did it start / how long has it been going on for?
- What were you doing at the time?

Clarify is this was a gradual change in breathing over several days or weeks or did it come on very rapidly over the space of hours or minutes? This will provide useful clues to the underlying cause.

Exacerbating and Relieving Factors
- Are you able to identify anything that triggers the breathlessness?
- Is there anything that makes the breathlessness better?

Is there something new, different or specific that causes the dyspnoea to start e.g. pets, perfume, dust, new medication, situations. Stopping an activity or doing something differently may provide clues.

Severity

- How bad would you say that your breathlessness is?

Can the patient speak in full sentences? Try to objectively quantify the breathlessness. The MRC dyspnoea scale is a useful tool (Table 3.3 below) to assess functional limitations.

Table 3.3 The Medical Research Council (MRC) dyspnoea scale [6]

Grade	Level of activity
1	Breathless during strenuous activity only
2	Breathless when hurrying or walking up a slight incline
3	Walking slower than peers due to breathlessness, or needs to pause for breath when walking at own pace
4	Pauses for breath after walking 100 m or a few minutes on level ground
5	Too breathless to leave the house, or breathless when dressing

Common Causes of Shortness of Breath [7]

Respiratory	Upper and lower respiratory tract infections,
	Obstructive and restrictive lung diseases,
	Upper airways obstruction
	Pulmonary embolus
Cardiac	Congestive cardiac failure, acute coronary syndromes, arrythmias.
MSK	Chest wall pain and trauma
Metabolic	Anaemia, sepsis, CO poisoning, acid-base imbalance
Psychological	Stress / anxiety / panic

Approach to Management

Dyspnoea is an uncomfortable, distressing experience. Calm and reassurance will help in all situations. Following a thorough history taking, a detailed cardio-respiratory examination is important to establish clinical signs and look for evidence of systemic disease / impacts elsewhere such as cyanosis, clubbing, oedema or calf swelling [5]. Check basic observations including blood pressure, pulse and oxygen saturations.

Blood tests	FBC, U&E's, inflammatory markers, clotting studies, Troponin if relevant, arterial blood gases.
Imaging	CXR
Other	ECG
	Peak expiratory flow rate (PEFR) and spirometry
	Well's score if considering PE
	ECHO if thought to be cardiac
Treatment	Nurse upright
	Oxygen if required (caution in COPD)
	Treat the underlying cause
	ICU input if ventilation is compromised or patient is haemodynamically unstable
Red flags	Sudden onset severe dyspnoea
	Tachypnoea >30 breaths per minute
	Impaired oxygen saturation
	Haemoptysis
	Marked weight loss
	Abnormal ECG
	Stridor (may indicate upper airways obstruction)
	Features of respiratory failure and use of accessory muscles
	Altered level of consciousness
	Cyanosis

COUGH = a sudden, forceful release of air to clear an irritation in the throat or airway [8]

Onset + Duration

- When did it start / how long has it been going on for?
- How frequent is this?
- Have you had previous episodes of a cough?

An acute cough is present for less than 3 weeks, sub-acute cough is present for 3–6 weeks and a chronic cough persists for more than 6–8 weeks.

Productive Cough

- Is the cough dry or do you bring anything up when you cough?
- Can you describe this?
- Can you show me your sputum?
- How much are you coughing up?

If the patient is producing sputum, then it is important to ask about the quantity (teaspoonful, egg cupful etc), the colour (green, white, yellow, clear) and the consistency (frothy, thick / purulent, thin). If you can see it for yourself and send a sample for testing all the better.

Haemoptysis

- Do you ever cough up any blood?
- Are there small specks of blood or a larger amount?
- Are there frank blood clots?
- What colour is the blood, is it fresh red, or darker?

Haemoptysis is a red flag symptom for more serious pathology such as lung cancer and it is important to quantify the amount and understand the type of bloody liquid that is being expectorated.

Exacerbating and Relieving Factors

- Is there anything that makes the cough better or worse?
- Have there been any changes in your environment recently?
- What is the pattern of the cough, is it better or worse at night?

Has anything changed in the patient's life recently, from new medication to a new cat? Clarify if there is any diurnal variation as this may give clues to the underlying cause e.g. asthma cough is worse at night.

Common Causes of Cough [9]

Respiratory	Respiratory tract infections, exacerbations of underlying lung disease
	Allergens / irritants, bronchiectasis, lung cancer, pulmonary fibrosis, pulmonary embolism.
	Parasitic infections, aspergillosis.
Cardiac	Mitral stenosis, congestive cardiac failure.
Clotting	Coagulopathies, anticoagulant medication.
Vasculitides	Goodpasture's syndrome, Wegener's granulomatosis.

Approach to Management

Cardiorespiratory examination followed by a full systems review will help to establish if this is purely pulmonary disease or not [10]. Smokers are at high risk of lung cancer as well as exacerbations of underlying chronic lung disease.

Blood tests	FBC, U&E's, inflammatory markers, clotting studies, Immunoglobulin status.
Imaging	CXR, CT chest
Other	Peak flow testing
	Sputum analysis; microscopy and culture
	Bronchoscopy
Treatment	Treat the underlying causes
	Antihistamines, steroids and decongestants for allergic reactions
	Antibiotics for bacterial infections
	Consider mucolytics in those with chronic purulent sputum
Red flags	Haemoptysis
	Smoker with a new cough (over age 45)
	Dysphagia
	Recurrent chest infections
	Hoarseness
	Systemic symptoms

WHEEZE = a high-pitched whistling sound associated with a blocked airway [11]

Onset + Duration

- When did it start and how long has it been going on for?

What is the chronicity of the wheeze and does it coincide with other respiratory symptoms.

Pattern

- Does the wheeze happen all the time or just on breathing in or out?

Being able to differentiate an inspiratory from an expiratory wheeze is useful to clarify some types of lung pathology.

Inspiratory suggests obstruction of larger airways collapsing as you breathe in.

Expiratory suggests lower airway obstruction and collapse as you breathe out.

Exacerbating and Relieving Factors

- Is there anything that makes the wheeze better or worse?
- Does using your inhaler help improve the situation?

Are there any identifiable situations or environmental factors that exacerbate the wheeze?

Find out which types of inhalers and nebulisers does the patient use, how many times and how long does it take to have an effect?

Common Causes of Wheeze [12]

Respiratory	Asthma, COPD, bronchitis, respiratory infections
	Pulmonary fibrosis, pulmonary oedema
	Foreign body aspiration
	Allergic reactions (anaphylaxis)
Cardiac	Congestive cardiac failure ('cardiac asthma')
GI	Gastro-oesophageal reflux disease
	Aspiration pneumonitis

Approach to Management

The examination and work up for wheeze are very similar to that for cough and dyspnoea. Serial peak flow measurements recorded over time can be useful to track response.

Treatment	Treat the underlying cause
	Trial of bronchodilators
	Humidified oxygen
Red flags	Features of respiratory distress
	Use of accessory muscles
	Silent chest
	Cyanosis
	Facial / tongue / mouth swelling

PLEURITIC CHEST PAIN / PLEURISY = sharp chest pain, usually on inspiration, caused by lung inflammation [13]

Character

- How would you best describe the type of pain that you are getting in your chest?
- Is it sharp, stabbing, heavy, burning?

Inflammation of the pleura causes sharp chest discomfort that is worsened by breathing and coughing.

Location

- Whereabouts are you getting the chest pain?
- Is the pain localised or diffuse?
- Does the pain spread anywhere?

Ask where specifically the pain is located and any radiation.

Onset + Duration

- When did it start / how long has it been going on for?
- Was it sudden onset or gradual?
- What were you doing when the pain started?

The timing of the pain can help signal the underlying cause. More gradual onset suggests a slow inflammatory process.

Exacerbating and Relieving Factors

- What makes the pain better or worse?
- Was there anything that you think might have triggered it?
- Have you experienced any recent trauma? Falls, fights, heavy lifting etc.

Deep breathing, lying flat and movement typically make pleuritic pain worse. Shallow breathing, sitting upright and analgesia tend to improve the situation.

Severity

- How bad is the pain on a scale of 1 to 10?

Understanding how bad the symptoms are helps to quantify and track the progression / resolution of any pains.

Common Causes of Pleuritic Chest Pain [14]

Respiratory	Pneumonia, Pulmonary embolism, Pneumothorax,
	Infections e.g. respiratory viruses, tuberculosis.
	Lung cancer.
Cardiac	Acute coronary syndromes, pericarditis
Musculoskeletal	Costochondritis, chest wall trauma, rheumatological conditions

Approach to Management

Cardio-respiratory examination and baseline observations including oxygen saturation and spirometry. Pleuritic chest pain typically worsens with deep breathing, coughing, or movement, and can indicate various conditions affecting the lungs, pleura, or chest wall [15].

Blood tests	FBC, U&E's, Inflammatory markers, clotting studies.
	D-dimers and / or Troponin where relevant.
	Arterial blood gas.
Imaging	CXR, CT chest, Chest wall ultrasound.
Treatment	Analgesia
	Oxygen if hypoxic
	Nurse upright
	Heat packs if available
	Folded blanket or cushion to act as a shock absorber
	Identify and treat the underlying cause.
Red flags	Sudden onset severe symptoms
	Haemodynamic instability
	Abnormal ECG

A Note on Spirometry

Interpreting FEV1 and FVC is essential in assessing lung function particularly in diagnosing and monitoring respiratory diseases such as **obstructive** and **restrictive lung diseases** [16].

FEV1: The amount of air a person can forcibly exhale in one second. It reflects the degree of airway obstruction.

FVC: The total volume of air that can be forcibly exhaled after taking the deepest breath possible. It assesses the full capacity of the lungs.

FEV1/FVC ratio: The proportion of air exhaled in the first second relative to the total amount exhaled. It helps distinguish between obstructive and restrictive patterns.

Normal FEV1/FVC ratio: Typically >70% (0.7) in adults, meaning at least 70% of the air can be expelled in the first second of forced expiration.

Low FEV1/FVC ratio: <70% suggests **airflow obstruction**, a hallmark of **obstructive lung diseases** like asthma or COPD.

Normal or high FEV1/FVC ratio with reduced lung volumes suggests a **restrictive lung pattern**.

INTERESTING FACT: If you unfolded both of your lungs, along with all the alveoli inside them, they would stretch out to the size of a tennis court. It is estimated that there are around 300–500 million alveoli in a pair of adult lungs [17].

References

1. Haddad M, Sharma S. Physiology, lung. In: StatPearls. Treasure Island (FL): StatPearls Publishing; 2023. Available from: https://www.ncbi.nlm.nih.gov/books/NBK545177/
2. Kuzniar, J. Assessment of dyspnoea. BMJ Best Practice; 2025. Available from: https://bestpractice.bmj.com/topics/en-gb/862
3. Kilgore D, Najm W. Common respiratory diseases. Prim Care. 2010;37(2):297–324.
4. Schaefer-Prokop C, Elicker BM. Pulmonary manifestations of systemic diseases. In: Hodler J, Kubik-Huch RA, von Schulthess GK, editors. Diseases of the chest, breast, heart and vessels 2019–2022: diagnostic and interventional imaging. Cham (CH): Springer; 2019. Chapter 11. Available from: https://www.ncbi.nlm.nih.gov/books/NBK553857/; https://doi.org/10.1007/978-3-030-11149-6_11
5. NICE. Breathlessness. clinical knowledge summary; 2024. Available from: https://cks.nice.org.uk/topics/breathlessness/references/
6. Williams N. The MRC breathlessness scale. Occup Med. 2017;67(6):496–7.
7. Sandberg J, Olsson M, Ekström M. Underlying conditions contributing to breathlessness in the population. Curr Opin Support Palliat Care. 2021;15(4):219–225.
8. McCrory DC, Coeytaux RR, Yancy WS Jr. Assessment and management of chronic cough. Rockville (MD): Agency for Healthcare Research and Quality (US); 2013 (Comparative Effectiveness Reviews, No. 100). Available from: https://www.ncbi.nlm.nih.gov/books/NBK116695/
9. Satia I, Wahab M, Kum E, Kim H, Lin P, Kaplan A, Field S. K. Chronic cough: investigations, management, current and future treatments. Can J Respir Crit Care Sleep Med. 2021;5(6): 404–416.
10. NICE. Cough: how should I assess a person with cough? 2025. Available from: https://cks.nice.org.uk/topics/cough/diagnosis/assessment/
11. Al-Shamrani A, Bagais K, Alenazi A, Alqwaiee M, Al-Harbi AS. Wheezing in children: approaches to diagnosis and management. Int J Pediatr Adolesc Med. 2019;6(2):68–73.
12. Mellis, C. Respiratory noises: how useful are they clinically? Pediatr Clin North Am. 2009; 56(1):1–17.
13. Reamy BV, Williams PM, Odom MR. Pleuritic chest pain: sorting through the differential diagnosis. Am Fam Physician. 2017;96(5):306–312.
14. Lee RW, Hodgson LE, Jackson MB, Adams N. Problem based review: pleuritic chest pain. Acute Med. 2012;11(3):172–82.
15. NICE Chest pain. Clinical knowledge summary; 2022. https://cks.nice.org.uk/topics/chest-pain/
16. Moore B Spirometry: step by step. Breathe. 2012;8(3):232–240.
17. Ananda Rao A, Johncy S. Tennis courts in the human body: a review of the misleading metaphor in medical literature. Cureus. 2022;14(1):e21474.

Chapter 4
The Gastroenterology System

Abstract The digestive system comprises everything from the mouth to the anus, and includes the liver, biliary tree, gallbladder and pancreas. It can give rise to a huge number of medical (and psychological) conditions, which in turn manifest themselves as disturbance in gut functioning and a variety of symptoms with a wide differential diagnosis. In this chapter we'll focus on what to ask when faced with abdominal pain, eructation and the like. The key condition that Gastroenterologists are arguably most interested in is bowel cancer as it remains a significant source of morbidity and mortality.

Keywords Nausea · Vomiting · Diarrhoea · Constipation · Abdominal pain · Altered bowel habit · Bowel cancer · Inflammatory bowel disease · Dysphagia · Gastro-oesophageal reflux disease

Introduction

Gastroenterology is a high demand speciality and there are a wide range of conditions that affect the gut. These tend to manifest in classic patterns, including nausea, vomiting, abdominal pain, change in bowel habit, reflux and rectal bleeding, and it is the job of the attentive clinician to decipher what it is going on. Table 4.1 summarises the common presenting complaints and Table 4.2 displays the commonest gastroenterological diseases and how they may be expressed.

Background History for the GI System

Several medical conditions affecting the GI system can run in families and a large number of dietary and environmental factors can play a part, so before you get started it's useful to establish the following [3].

P. Grant, *The Concise Guide to Medical History Taking*,
https://doi.org/10.1007/978-3-031-91474-4_4

Table 4.1 Summary table of presenting GI complaints and differential diagnoses [1]

GI system presenting complaints	Commonly associated conditions
Abdominal pain	Location matters **Epigastric area:** suggests cardiac and gastric issues but also gall bladder disease and pancreatitis **Right upper quadrant:** hepato-biliary disease, renal disease **Left upper quadrant:** pancreatic disease, renal disease, cardiac **Periumbilical:** gastric disease, vascular pathology, colonic/early appendicitis **Right lower quadrant:** colonic disease e.g. colitis. Gynae disease, renal disease **Left lower quadrant:** gynae disease e.g. uterine fibroids. Renal disease **Supra-pubic:** cystitis, nephrolithiasis, diverticulitis, IBD, IBS, uterine fibroids, ovarian mass, torsion **Non-specific:** bowel obstruction, mesenteric ischaemia, peritonitis, IBD, sickle cell crisis **Abdominal wall:** muscle strain, herpes zoster, hernias
Abdominal distension	The 5 "F's" – fat, fluid, flatus, foetus and faeces
Change in bowel habit	Bowel cancer, inflammatory bowel disease, irritable bowel syndrome, diverticular disease
Constipation	Dehydration, sub-optimal diet, medication side effects, immobility, intestinal obstruction, metabolic disorders
Diarrhoea	Infective causes, IBS, IBD, bowel cancer, medication side effects, coeliac disease
Dysphagia	Mechanical blockage e.g. Oesophageal cancer. Oesophagitis secondary to GORD, motility problems due to achalasia or neurological disorders
Indigestion	Gastro-oesophageal reflux disease, obesity, hiatus hernia, smoking, pregnancy, stress and anxiety, medications e.g. NSAIDs
Nausea / vomiting	Gastroenteritis, intestinal obstruction, medication side effects, metabolic disorders, neurological disorders, psychiatric
Burping (eructation)	Aerophagia, Gastritis/GORD, dietary factors
Jaundice	Liver failure, Hepatitis, Haemolysis, Alcoholic liver disease, Liver cirrhosis, Gallstones, Pancreatitis, Malignancy
Rectal bleeding	Anal disorders such as haemorrhoids, bowel cancer, inflammatory bowel disease, diverticulitis, gastroenteritis
Malaena	Upper GI bleed, but don't forget exogenous influences such as beetroot, Guinness and iron tablets

Table 4.2 Summary table of common GI conditions and associated symptoms [2]

Common GI conditions	Common symptoms
Coeliac disease	Weight loss, abdominal pains and bloating, diarrhoea, fatigue, steatorrhoea, nausea and vomiting
Inflammatory bowel disease e.g. Crohn's / UC	Weight loss, abdominal cramps/pains, change in bowel habit, rectal bleeding, weight loss, pyrexia, oral ulceration, passing mucous PR, increased bowel opening frequency, tenesmus
Liver failure	Jaundice, confusion, drowsiness, neurological features such as asterixis (jumpy movements)
Irritable bowel syndrome	Change in bowel habit/excitable, abdominal pains and bloating (often improved after emptying bowels), tenesmus, stress
Hepatitis	Jaundice, ascites, fever, malaise
Bowel cancer	Change in bowel habit, rectal bleeding, abdominal distension and pain, weight loss, fatigue
Gastro-oesophageal reflux disease	Epigastric and chest pain, acid reflux symptoms / heartburn, swallowing problems, burping
Pancreatitis	Epigastric pain, weight loss, hyperosmolar symptoms
Gallstones	Jaundice, abdominal pain (RUQ and epigastric), pruritus

- History of previous medical or surgical problems affecting the GI system or liver and any previous investigations such as endoscopies or operations such as laparotomies?
- Do they have a family history of any GI conditions, (especially IBD, FAP and bowel cancer as these have a genetic component)?
- Medications—multiple drugs, both prescribed and recreational, as well as alcohol can impact the gut. Make sure that you get a full list of what they are taking.
- Constitutional upset—have you lost any weight recently? Have your diet or eating patterns changed? What is your normal bowel habit?
- Alcohol history—this is very relevant to GI conditions such as liver disease, peptic ulcer disease and pancreatitis.

CONSTIPATION = difficulty to pass stool [4]

Onset + Duration
- When did it start / how long has it been going on for?

The longer the duration the more serious the complaint is likely to be and the more difficult to treat.

Frequency of Bowel Opening
- How often are you able to open your bowels successfully (per day / week etc)?

Obtain quantifiable information as this can guide response to treatment.

What's Normal
- When things are normal how regularly do you open your bowels?
- How would you describe your stools?

Knowing the baseline can indicate the severity of the constipation.

Stool Type
- How would you describe your stools?

Are we talking small hard pellets or large normal bowel motions followed by large amounts of liquid stool. You will get used to the amount of detail that people are happy to go into.

Rectal Bleeding
- Is there any blood in your stools, and if so tell me more?

The colour and relationship of blood in the stools is suggestive of the underlying pathology. Red blood mixed in with the stools indicates colorectal lesions such as IBD, cancer and diverticular disease. Bright red blood on the surface of the stool or on the toilet tissue suggests rectosigmoid disease e.g. haemorrhoids. Altered blood or clots is always an alarm sign for serious disease such as colorectal cancer or IBD.

Mucous
- Is there any slime or mucous in your stools?

The presence of mucous is abnormal and can represent infection, inflammation such as with IBD or proctitis and IBS.

Ano-Rectal Issues
- Do you experience anal pain related to opening your bowels and do you ever feel that you haven't completely evacuated your bowels?

Anal pain from trauma, rectal abscesses or haemorrhoids can exacerbate constipation. The feeling of incomplete bowel emptying is known as 'tenesmus' and is associated with a range of GI conditions from motility disorders to IBD.

Common Causes of Constipation [4]

GI	Dietary factors e.g. low fibre intake, dairy products, processed food.
	Structural disorders e.g. bowel strictures, bowel cancer, rectocoele.
	Diverticular disease. Irritable bowel syndrome.
	Dehydration.
Metabolic	Hypothyroidism, poorly controlled Diabetes, Hypercalcaemia, Hypokalaemia, Pregnancy.
Neurological	Parkinson's disease, Multiple sclerosis, Spinal cord injury, Stroke.
Psychological	Depression, stress, anxiety, eating disorders, functional disorders.
MSK	Pelvic floor dysfunction, immobility, post-surgery.
Medication	Calcium channel blockers, diuretics, beta-blockers, opiates, anti-histamines, anti-depressants, anti-cholinergics.

Approach to Management

Abdominal examination is useful to assess whether there is an abdominal mass or faecal impaction. Don't forget a rectal examination to both inspect the anus and feel for any blockages or tumours.

Blood tests	FBC to check for anaemia, Iron studies,
	U&E's to assess for renal impairment and dehydration
	Electrolytes e.g. hypercalcaemia, hypokalaemia
	Inflammatory markers
	TFT's to consider hypothyroidism
Imaging	Plain abdominal X-ray or a CT scan may be indicated.
	Lower GI endoscopy, barium enema can be performed if there is a suspicion of malignancy. Taking a biopsy can diagnose colitis.
Treatment	Try to manage the underlying cause and if appropriate make sure that the patient is well hydrated.
	Mobilisation and dietary fibre really help including foodstuffs such as kiwifruit and prunes.
	Laxatives and stool softening agents are useful, followed by enemas if no improvement.
Red flags	Rectal bleeding and weight loss suggest malignancy.

DIARRHOEA = increased stool frequency, generally with increased liquidity [5]

Onset + Duration
- When did it start / how long has it been going on for?

Acute diarrhoea suggests an infective cause, chronic diarrhoea which alternates with constipation hints at IBS-M.

Frequency of Bowel Opening
- How often are you opening your bowels (per day / week etc)?

Obtain quantifiable information as this can guide response to treatment.

What's Normal
- When things are normal how regularly do you open your bowels?

Knowing the baseline can indicate the severity of the diarrhoea.

Stool Type
- How would you describe the consistency of your stools?

Are we talking large amounts of liquid stool or frequent normal stools.

Bloody Diarrhoea
- Do you get any blood in your stools or bleeding from the back passage?

The colour and relationship of blood in the stools is suggestive of the underlying pathology. Red blood mixed in with the stools indicates colorectal lesions such as IBD, cancer and diverticular disease. Bright red blood on the surface of the stool or on the toilet tissue suggests rectosigmoid disease e.g. haemorrhoids. Altered blood or clots is always an alarm sign for serious disease such as colorectal cancer or IBD.

Mucous
- Is there any pus, slime or mucous in your stools?

The presence of mucous is abnormal and can represent infection, polyps and inflammation such as with IBD or proctitis and IBS.

Environmental Exposure
- Have you travelled abroad recently or eaten anything new or different?
- Has anyone in your family or social circle been experiencing diarrhoea recently?

Traveller's diarrhoea is not uncommon when coming into contact with new 'foreign' viruses and bacteria. Close contacts suggest local transmission and an infective cause.

Common Causes of Diarrhoea [6]

GI	Malabsorption e.g. Coeliac disease, lactose intolerance, short bowel syndrome (post-op). Inflammatory bowel disease, Diverticulitis.
	Colo-rectal cancer.
	Hepato-biliary disease e.g. chronic liver disease, post cholecystecomy, primary sclerosing cholangitis.
Dietary	Alcohol, high fat diet, artificial sweeteners.
Metabolic	Hyperthyroidism, poorly controlled Diabetes, Carcionoid syndrome (rare), Zollinger-Ellison syndrome (rare). Cystic fibrosis.
Infections	Bacterial infections: e.g. Salmonella, Shigella, Campylobacter, E. coli, Clostridium difficile, Vibrio cholerae.
	Viral infections: e.g. Norovirus, Rotavirus, Adenovirus, Hepatitis A.
	Parasitic infections: e.g. Giardia lamblia, Entamoeba histolytica, Cryptosporidium, Strongyloides.
Neurological	Autonomic neuropathy e.g. Parkinson's disease, diabetes.
	Stroke or spinal cord injury.
Psychological	Irritable bowel syndrome. Stress and anxiety.
Medications	Laxatives, antibiotics, Metformin, NSAIDs, PPI's, chemotherapy.

Approach to Management

Assess the patient to see if they look otherwise unwell e.g. have lost weight or appear dehydrated or anaemic. Don't forget an abdominal examination to feel for masses and a rectal examination to both inspect the anus and feel for any blockages or tumours [7].

Blood tests	FBC and Iron studies to check for anaemia, Inflammatory markers, U&E's to test for acute renal impairment.
	Full TFT's are useful and consider coeliac screening if the history suggests a relationship with certain food types.
Stool tests	Samples can be analysed for specific toxins, parasites, ova, occult blood, and newer tests such as faecal elastase and calprotectin can indicate GI inflammation. FIT test assesses for GI bleeding.
Imaging	Rigid or flexible sigmoidoscopy and colonoscopy can be a good way of visualising the gut and taking biopsies (assess for colitis).
	Barium enema can be useful for ruling out colorectal cancer and abdominal CT scanning can provide a helpful overview.
Treatment	Rehydration is an important consideration because of the risk of acute kidney injury, followed by treating the underlying cause and then considering anti-diarrhoeal agents such as loperamide or codeine.
	If an infective cause is suspected, the recommendation is to let the diarrhoea run its course.
	Antibiotics are indicated in cases of clostridium difficile related diarrhoea and best to discuss with the local microbiology team.
Red flags	Bloody diarrhoea with or without weight loss indicates serious pathology and needs to be worked up thoroughly.

DYSPHAGIA = difficulty in swallowing [8]

Onset + Duration
- When did it start / how long has it been going on for?

Progressive worsening over weeks to months suggests an oesophageal malignancy. An oesophageal ring can present intermittently.

Globus can be present for a prolonged period of time but with no other systemic upset.

Circumstances
- Does the difficulty in swallowing affect both solid foods as well as liquids?

If both are affected then a motility or upper GI (pharyngeal) problem is most likely. If the problem starts with solids and then liquids then the development of a stricture is likely.

Odynophagia
- Is it painful to swallow?

Indicates either severe GORD, malignancy, achalasia or oesophageal spasm.

Difficulty Initiating Swallowing
- Do you get any coughing, choking or regurgitation?

This suggests an oropharyngeal lesion or a bulbar palsy.

Risk Factors
- Are you a smoker or drink much alcohol?
- Have you previously suffered with indigestion / heartburn symptoms?
- Have you lost any weight recently?

The responses provide clues to underlying malignancy. It is important to quantify any weight loss / change in dress size / loose clothing.

Common Causes of Dysphagia [9]

GI	Mechanical blockage e.g. Oesophageal cancer. Pharyngeal pouch.
	Oesophagitis secondary to GORD, oesophageal strictures / webs.
	Foreign bodies causing obstruction.
	Motility problems due to achalasia, diffuse oesophageal spasm.
	Hiatus hernia.
Neurological	Stroke, Parkinson's disease, Multiple sclerosis.
Infections	Candida oesophagitis, HSV, CMV.
Rheumatological	Systemic sclerosis, Sjogren's syndrome, SLE.
Medications	Bisphosphonates, anti-cholinergics, NSAID's.
Psychological	Globus / functional, anxiety.

Approach to Management

Examine for any features of chronic liver disease, anaemia, malnutrition and lymphadenopathy. Look for features of any systemic illness, weight loss, malignancy.

Blood tests	FBC to test for anaemia, U&E's to assess for dehydration and AKI, Inflammatory markers.
Imaging	Barium swallow or upper GI endoscopy depending on local guidelines.
Treatment	Identify and treat the underlying cause
	ENT review if oropharyngeal cause suspected, Speech therapist assessment to assist with practicalities of swallowing, Dietician review.
Red flags	Odynophagia, Constant and worsening or complete dysphagia.

DYSPEPSIA = acid reflux / heartburn / indigestion [10]

Onset + Duration
- When did it start / how long has it been going on for?
- How often do you experience this problem?

The time course can provide information about the likely underlying cause. Symptoms that rapidly progress are more concerning.

Exacerbating and Relieving Factors
- Does anything make the acid reflux / indigestion problems worse or helps things improve?
- Does the discomfort change when changing position ie. leaning forwards or lying down?

There may be certain foods or drinks that contribute.
Positional changes give clues to the aetiology, lying down suggests GORD whereas improvement on leaning forward suggests pericarditis.

Self-Management
- What treatments have you tried?

Gaviscon commonly works well for GORD, as do PPI medications, but they won't make a difference with non-ulcer dyspepsia.

Associated Symptoms
- Do you ever experience any food coming back up into your mouth?
- Do you tend to feel full up quickly?
- Do you have any symptoms such as weakness, lethargy or shortness of breath?
- Have you had episodes of vomiting up blood or passing very dark stools?

Regurgitation suggests an oropharyngeal issue such as a pouch or an obstructive lesion.
Early satiety is suggestive of a gastric malignancy. Asking specifically about symptoms of iron deficiency anaemia is useful. Evidence of haematemesis or melaena is a red flag.

Common Causes of Dyspepsia [11]

GI	Oesophagitis, gastro-oesophageal reflux disease, gastric malignancy, peptic/ duodenal ulcer disease, non-ulcer dyspepsia.
	Hiatus hernia, oesophageal cancer, gastroparesis.
	Hepato-biliary disease. Pancreatitis.
Infections	Viral gastroenteritis, H. Pylori infection, Giardiasis, Amoebiasis.
Metabolic	Poorly controlled diabetes, hypercalcaemia, thyroid disorders.
Psychological	Stress, anxiety.
Medications	NSAID's, antibiotics, iron tablets, alcohol, steroids.
Other	Obesity, pregnancy, food intolerances

Approach to Management

It's important to rule out cardiac issues as dyspepsia associated epigastric pain for example may be cardiac in origin. Patients with significant indigestion related problems need dietary and lifestyle advice along with anti-acid treatments. If there are any worrying symptoms that suggest malignancy, then they require urgent investigation and diagnosis [12].

Blood tests	FBC to check for iron deficiency anaemia, Fe studies and haematinics.
	U&E's, LFT's, Amylase.
	Inflammatory markers.
	Electrolytes including calcium.
	HbA1c, TFT's.
Imaging	Barium swallow, upper GI endoscopy, abdominal CT scanning.
Other	H.Pylori testing and consider oesophageal manometry and pH studies.
Treatment	Lifestyle advice
	Anti-acid therapy for symptoms
	Eradication treatment for H. Pylori infection.
	Treat the underlying cause wherever possible.
Red flags	Weight loss, iron deficiency anaemia, rapid onset and progression of symptoms, dysphagia, upper GI bleeding.

ABDOMINAL PAIN = pain in the abdomen can be a manifestation of multiple conditions in the surgical sieve affecting individual organs, the peritoneum and mesentery, as well as non-gut metabolic conditions and pain referred from elsewhere in the body [12]

Location
- Whereabouts are you getting the abdominal pain, and does it spread anywhere?

Different disease processes relate to different areas;

Foregut pain (stomach) localises to the gastric area.

Liver and gallbladder problems affect the right upper quadrant.

Midgut pain manifests in the periumbilical area.

Hindgut pain is expressed in the suprapubic region.

Ureteric pain radiates from 'loin to groin'.

Gallbladder pain can be referred to the tip of the right scapula and diaphragmatic pain can be referred to the right shoulder.

Onset + Duration
- When did it start / how long has it been going on for?

Sudden onset abdominal pain indicates a vascular event or the perforation of a viscus.

Character
- How best would you describe the type of pain that you are getting?

Intermittent pain suggests colic, whereas constant pain indicates peritoneal involvement.

Severity
- How bad would you rate the severity of your pain out of 10 (if 10 is the worst pain ever)?

Gives a very good indication of how significant the problem is but is also a useful marker of change / improvement.

Exacerbating and Relieving Factors
- Does anything make the pain better or worse?

Movement can trigger peritonitis to worsen so patients tend to lie still.

Colicky pain can make patients restless and move about a lot.

Eating certain (fatty) foods can cause gallbladder pain.

Pain from pancreatitis or GORD can be relieved by sitting forwards.

Associated Issues
- Any history of trauma? Rule out any obvious injuries.
- Change in bowel habit? Likely relates to gut disease.
- Any swelling of the abdomen?
- When was you last period?
- Have you lost any weight recently?
- Do you have urinary problems?

- Have you had a high temperature?
- Any nausea or vomiting?

Rule out any obvious injuries. With an acute abdomen distension can be related to fluid, gas, fibroids and faecal impaction. In women of childbearing age, make sure to ask about menstrual irregularity, pregnancy and vaginal discharge as it may be a gynaecological issue. Could this be an ectopic pregnancy?

Chronic weight loss is suggestive of an underlying malignancy. Urinary symptoms such as dysuria and frequency can indicate urological disorders. The presence of pyrexia suggests and infective cause such as gastroenteritis or appendicitis. Establish the nature and frequency of any vomiting.

Common Causes of Abdominal Pain by Location [3]

Epigastric	Cardiac disease, GORD, gastric ulcer, pancreatitis.
Right upper quadrant	Hepatobiliary disease, duodenal ulcer, right lower lobe pneumonia.
Right lower quadrant	Appendicitis, renal colic, inflammatory bowel disease, diverticulitis, psoas abscess, strangulated hernia.
Umbilical	Pancreatitis, appendicitis, ruptured aortic aneurysm, diverticulitis.
Left upper quadrant	GORD, gastric ulcer disease, splenic rupture, left lower lobe pneumonia.
Left lower quadrant	Diverticular disease, colonic perforation, inflammatory bowel disease, renal colic, strangulated hernia.
Abdominal wall	Muscle strain, herpes zoster, hernias.
Generalised	Bowel obstruction, mesenteric ischaemia, peritonitis, IBD, sickle cell crisis.

Approach to Management

Abdominal examination is vital to assess the site of discomfort and whether there is an abdominal mass [13, 14]. Don't forget a rectal examination. Monitor vital signs and be wary of hypotension and tachycardia. Get an ECG to rule out cardiac issues.

Blood tests	FBC to check for anaemia, LFT's to assess liver status, U&E's to rule out AKI, ESR and CRP to test for inflammation, Amylase to consider pancreatitis, Arterial blood gas to assess overall condition / acidosis.
	Blood cultures if likely sepsis.
	Urinalysis to check for infection.
Imaging	AXR, Abdominal ultrasound, CT scanning, Laparoscopy
Treatment	Provide analgesia—don't worry about 'masking' pain, IV fluids for dehydration and resuscitation.
	Treat the underlying cause.
	Early referral to helpful surgeons.
Red flags	Sudden onset severe pain, weight loss.

NAUSEA & VOMITING = feeling or being sick, a very common and troubling complaint [15, 16]

Onset + Duration
- When did it start / how long has it been going on for?

Timeframe and progression is useful. Clarify relationship to potential precipitants.

Timing / Precipitants
- Is there any particular time of day when you experience this problem or is there anything that you can identify which triggers the nausea / vomiting?

The timing and relationship to food intake are very useful pieces of information. Additionally, are there other factors / activities that precede the vomiting?

Quantity
- How much are you vomiting each time?

The quantity provides clues e.g. a small amount is more likely to be an oropharyngeal problem, as opposed to a larger amount—full stomach contents.

Characterisation
- Can you describe the vomit?

Clarify if they have true haematemesis. What the vomit looks like is useful to know; solids or liquids, bile containing, bloody, coffee grounds, contains faeces etc.

Associated Symptoms
- Have you lost any weight?
- Have you lost your appetite?
- Are you experiencing any abdominal pains?
- Any change in bowel habit?
- Any recent foreign travel?
- Any close contacts who've also been unwell?
- What treatments have you tried?

Weight loss and anorexia are suggestive of an underlying malignancy. GI upset is covered in the section above. Consider infective causes and find out if the patient has managed to find anything to settle the symptoms.

Common Causes of Nausea and Vomiting [16]

GI	Gastroenteritis, intestinal obstruction, pancreatitis, cholecystitis, paralytic ileus.
Metabolic disease	DKA, AKI / uraemia, high calcium, low sodium.
Neurological	Raised intracranial pressure, labyrinthitis, migraine, meningitis.
Other	Don't forget pregnancy, alcohol, drugs, infective illnesses, MI, psychogenic.

Approach to Management

Patients with vomiting are at high risk of fluid and electrolyte loss. Assess for dehydration and ensure that you have a full set of observations including blood pressure and temperature [16]. Monitoring fluid input and output is sensible. Abdominal examination will help identify GI pathology such as obstruction.

Blood tests	FBC, LFT's, U&E's to rule out AKI.
	Amylase and corrected calcium.
	ABG to assess degree of compromise.
Imaging	AXR can help to rule out bowel obstruction.
	OGD if vomiting is persistent.
Treatment	Try to manage the underlying cause, PO/IV rehydration, Anti-emetics, Monitor renal function and electrolytes.
Red flags	Weight loss, coffee ground vomiting, haematemesis, dehydration.

JAUNDICE = yellowing of the skin and eyes due to the deposition of bilirubin [17]

Onset + Duration
- When do you think that the jaundice started?
- How long has it been going on for?
- Is the jaundice present all the time or does it come and go?

Gradual development suggests insidious liver disease. Sudden onset suggests acute liver failure or other acute illnesses. If the jaundice is intermittent, then it may be due to a transient cause such as Gilbert's syndrome.

Precipitants
- Any recent illnesses or surgery?

Infective illnesses such as Mycoplasma and some general anaesthetic agents such as Halothane can cause jaundice.

Associations
- Is the jaundice associated with any of the following; dark urine colour, change in the colour of your stool, itchiness?
- Have you been experiencing any abdominal pain?

The presence of pruritus, dark urine (urobilin) and discoloured stools (stercobilin) supports the findings of jaundice. In the context of abdominal pain jaundice may be due to cholecystitis, pancreatitis or pancreatic cancer.

Risk Factors for Hepatitis
Are any of the following applicable to you;

- Close contact with someone who has a diagnosis of Hepatitis?
- Recent foreign travel?
- Any immune disorders?
- Have you ever injected drugs, tattoos?
- Blood transfusions in a foreign country?

Viral forms of hepatitis A/B/C should be considered.

Neurological Features
- Any recent confusion, tremors, slurred speech, forgetfulness, personality changes.

Neurological issues are suggestive of hepatic encephalopathy or EtOH withdrawal.

Common Causes of Jaundice [18]

Pre-hepatic	Haemolysis, Gilbert's syndrome, thalassaemia, sickle cell anaemia, Glucose-6-Phosphate deficiency.
Liver disease	Viral hepatitis, Alcoholic liver disease / cirrhosis due to any cause, primary or secondary liver malignancies.
Post-hepatic	Cholestasis, pancreatic mass, biliary disease.
Congenital / inherited	Wilson's disease, Alpha-1 antitrypsin deficiency.
Other	Alcohol, drugs e.g. all drugs.

Approach to Management

A thorough history is required to try and tease apart the potential aetiology [17]. Abdominal examination and liver palpation is useful. Look for signs of malignancy and features of chronic liver disease. Broad systems enquiry.

Blood tests	LFT's, albumin, clotting, gamma GT, FBC, blood film, U&E's, amylase. ABG.
Imaging	Liver ultrasound, ERCP / MRCP, abdominal CT
Treatment	Manage the underlying condition. Remove any potential precipitants. Stop alcohol. Chlordiazepoxide if withdrawal. Refer to the liver specialists
Red flags	Weight loss, neurological features, very abnormal LFT's.

MALAENA = dark, tarry, offensive stools, suggestive of an upper GI bleed [19]

Onset + Duration
- When did it start / how long has it been going on for?
  Duration is important as if prolonged anaemia is more likely.

Amount and Frequency
- How would you describe your stools, how much do you produce each time and how often has it been occurring?

Are the classic malaena stools being described or is it more related to bright red / blood mixed in with the stools which are suggestive of lower GI or ano-rectal pathology.

Precipitants
- Was there anything that happened before you experienced this problem?

Find out if there was a significant amount of vomiting ie. to induce a Mallory-Weiss tear?

A recent alcohol binge? Also ask about new medications e.g. NSAIDs?

Anaemia Symptoms
- Specifically, have you any of the following, lethargy, breathlessness, angina, light-headedness or confusion?

Anaemia is common following malaena and can manifest in a variety of ways.

Associated Symptoms
- Any abdominal pain?
- Any symptoms of indigestion?
- Do you get full easily?

Consider location as a clue to underlying causes.
Could the malaena be due to upper GI bleeding?
Early satiety is a sign suggestive of gastric malignancy.

Features of Potential Hypotension
- Have you been feeling faint?
- Tired?
- Palpitations?
- Confusion?

These can signify potential haemodynamic instability after an episode of GI bleeding.

Common Causes of Melaena [20]

GI	Oesophageal varices, Mallory-Weiss tear,
	GORD—oesophagitis / duodenitis / gastritis, peptic ulceration, H.Pylori.
	Gastric, oesophageal or small bowel malignancy.
	Angiodysplasia
	Trauma to the GI tract, post GI surgery or endoscopy.
Medications	Drugs such as aspirin, NSAID's, steroids, anticoagulants.

Approach to Management

Ensure you have IV access and send bloods early for FBC and cross match as a transfusion may be required. Abdominal examination with a PR is essential. Look for signs of chronic liver disease. Assess the patient's haemodynamic status and GCS. Monitor fluid input and output. Keep patient NBM [20].

Blood tests	FBC, clotting studies, blood film, cross match and group and save.
	LFT's, U&E's, Amylase, Inflammatory markers.
Imaging	Calculate the Rockall score and discuss the urgency of an upper GI endoscopy.
Treatment	IV access, fluid resuscitate, NG tube if required.
	Correct clotting abnormalities.
	Manage the underlying cause and consider PPI therapy post endoscopy.
Red flags	Anaemia, weight loss, haemodynamic instability, early satiety.

INTERESTING FACT: The gut is home to tens of millions of microscopic organisms. There are more than 100 billion bacteria to every gram of intestinal content. Almost half the dry weight of human faeces is made up of E.Coli bacteria [21].

References

1. Approaches and chief complaints in gastroenterology. In: Huppert LA, Dyster TG, editors. Huppert's notes: pathophysiology and clinical pearls for internal medicine. McGraw Hill; 2021.
2. Jabłońska B, Mrowiec S. Gastrointestinal disease: new diagnostic and therapeutic approaches. Biomedicines. 2023;11(5):1420.
3. Boston University Medical Campus. Guidelines for the history and physical exam write up. 2008. https://www.google.com/url?sa=t&source=web&rct=j&opi=89978449&url=https:// www.bumc.bu.edu/im-residency/files/2010/10/History-and-Physical-Exam-Guidelines. doc&ved=2ahUKEwjgyP_omtqKAxWKVkEAHflROBMQFnoECA8QAQ&usg=AOvVaw0 7I71yo6enbX_-NMb7msAN. Accessed 23 June 2024.

4. Diaz S, Bittar K, Hashmi MF, et al. Constipation. [Updated 2023 Nov 12]. In: StatPearls [Internet]. Treasure Island (FL): StatPearls; 2025 Jan. https://www.ncbi.nlm.nih.gov/books/NBK513291/. Accessed 23 May 2024.

5. National Institute for Health and Care Excellence. Clinical knowledge summary. Constipation. 2024. https://cks.nice.org.uk/topics/constipation/. Accessed 1 May 2024.

6. National Institute for Health and Care Excellence. Clinical knowledge summary. Diarrhoea – adult's assessment. 2024. https://cks.nice.org.uk/topics/diarrhoea-adults-assessment/. Accessed 1 May 2024.

7. BMJ Best Practice. Assessment of chronic diarrhoea. BMJ Publishing Group; 2023b. http://bestpractice.bmj.com

8. Wilkinson JM, Codipilly DC, Wilfahrt RP. Dysphagia: evaluation and collaborative management. Am Fam Physician. 2021;103(2):97–106. PMID: 33448766.

9. Ahmed I, Matull R. Swallowing difficulties (dysphagia). In: Haydock S, Whitehead D, Fritz Z, editors. Acute medicine: a symptom-based approach. Cambridge University Press; 2014. p. 421–7.

10. National Institute for Health and Care Excellence. Clinical knowledge summary. Dyspepsia – unidentified cause. 2024. https://cks.nice.org.uk/topics/dyspepsia-unidentified-cause/. Accessed 21 May 2024.

11. Harmon RC, Peura DA. Evaluation and management of dyspepsia. Ther Adv Gastroenterol. 2010;3(2):87–98.

12. Malone M. Managing dyspepsia. J Fam Pract. 2015;64(6):350–7.

13. Sherman R. Chapter 86: abdominal pain. In: Walker HK, Hall WD, Hurst JW, editors. Clinical methods: the history, physical, and laboratory examinations. 3rd ed. Boston: Butterworths; 1990.

14. Cartwright SL, Knudson MP. Evaluation of acute abdominal pain in adults. Am Fam Physician. 2008;77(7):971–8. PMID: 18441863.

15. Scorza K, Williams A, Phillips JD, Shaw J. Evaluation of nausea and vomiting. Am Fam Physician. 2007;76(1):76–84. PMID: 17568843.

16. BMJ Best Practice. Assessment of nauseas and vomiting, adults. 2024. https://bestpractice.bmj.com/topics/en-gb/631. Accessed 21 May 2024.

17. National Institute for Health and Care Excellence. Clinical knowledge summary. Jaundice in adults. 2020. https://cks.nice.org.uk/topics/jaundice-in-adults/. Accessed 11 May 2024.

18. Fargo MV, Grogan SP, Saguil A. Evaluation of jaundice in adults. Am Fam Physician. 2017;95(3):164–8.

19. Minto M, Hollingworth TW. Haematemesis and melaena. Medicine. 2021;49(2):98–102. ISSN 1357-3039.

20. National Institute for Health and Care Excellence. Acute upper gastrointestinal bleeding in over 16s: management. Clinical guideline [CG141]. 2016. https://www.nice.org.uk/guidance/cg141. Accessed 9 Dec 2024.

21. van Houte J, Gibbons RJ. Studies of the cultivable flora of normal human feces. Antonie Van Leeuwenhoek. 1966;32(1):212–22. p.220.

Chapter 5
The Endocrine System

Abstract A hormone is a chemical messenger, released from one part of the body, travelling to an often-distant location to deliver instructions elsewhere in a very targeted manner. The endocrine system comprises multiple glands including the anterior and posterior pituitary (which together comprise the 'master gland'), the thyroid, the parathyroids, the adrenals, the kidney, the heart, the pancreas, and the gonads.

These glands can be hit by anything in the surgical sieve from haemorrhage, infection, and malignancy, through to an autoimmune attack. Disease often manifests in terms of patterns of hypo- or hyper-function of particular hormones and subsequently treatment of endocrine disease is often based around managing the replacement of a deficient hormone e.g. insulin in diabetes, or suppression of an overactive hormone e.g. using anti-thyroid medication in the context of thyrotoxicosis.

The expert Endocrinologist is able to identify the gestalt of such patterns and interpret the appropriate dynamic tests to elucidate the underlying problem. In this chapter we'll focus on what to ask when faced with symptoms of endocrine gland dysfunction. Many of these diseases are subtle and insidious so special attention needs to be paid by the discerning medical historian.

Keywords Thyroid disease · Diabetes mellitus · Hyperosmolar symptoms · Goitre · Menstrual disturbance · Galactorrhoea · Hirsutism · Fatigue · Erectile dysfunction

Introduction

The Endocrinologist is like a detective, piecing together clues and then tying the molecular mutations together with a set of clinical symptoms. Many hormonal disorders can manifest in subtle and insidious ways and it's important to know what to ask in the right way and at the right time. Table 5.1 summarises common presenting

P. Grant, *The Concise Guide to Medical History Taking*,
https://doi.org/10.1007/978-3-031-91474-4_5

Table 5.1 Summary table of Endocrine presenting complaints and differential diagnoses [1]

Endocrine system presenting complaints	Commonly associated conditions
Goitre	A goitre is an enlargement of the thyroid gland. Hypothyroidism, Grave's disease, Thyroid nodules, Thyroiditis, Pregnancy and Puberty.
Fatigue	Fatigue is a common symptom that can be associated with a variety of medical conditions across different systems of the body. Anaemia, diabetes, thyroid disorders, sleep disorders, depression and anxiety, malignancy, renal disease, COPD, medications.
Galactorrhoea	Hyperprolactinaemia, hypothyroidism, Polycystic Ovarian Syndrome (PCOS), medications including anti-psychotics and anti-depressants. Chest wall stimulation. Pregnancy.
Gynaecomastia	Puberty, ageing, hypogonadism, liver disease, kidney failure, thyroid disorders, tumours of the testes, adrenal glands, or pituitary. Medications including anti-androgens, anabolic steroids, anti-depressants. Alcohol and narcotics e.g. cannabis.
Menstrual disturbance	PCOS, Thyroid disorders, Endometriosis, Fibroids, Peri-menopause, Stress, heavy exercise, Eating disorders, Pregnancy, Hyperprolactinaemia, Primary ovarian insufficiency.
Hirsutism	PCOS, Congenital adrenal hyperplasia (CAH), Cushing's syndrome, Androgen secreting tumours, Hypothyroidism, Medications including anabolic steroids or Danazol. Insulin resistance.
Thyroid hormone dysfunction	Signs of metabolic over or underactivity due to thyroiditis, autoimmune conditions, pituitary disorders and medications such as Amiodarone.
Erectile dysfunction	Hypogonadism, diabetes, obesity, cardiovascular disease / atherosclerosis, hypertension, neurological disorders, psychological disorders including depression. Medications including anti-depressants. Alcohol and narcotics e.g. cannabis.
Polydipsia / polyuria	Diabetes mellitus, Diabetes insipidus, Primary (psychogenic) polydipsia, Hypercalcaemia, renal disease, liver disease Medications including diuretics, calcium channel blockers, lithium. Pregnancy.
Hypoglycaemia / hyperglycaemia	Diabetes mellitus, Insulin resistances, Cushing's syndrome, Acromegaly, Pancreatitis, Phaeochromocytoma, Adreno-cortical insufficiency. Medications including sulphonylureas, insulin, steroids, phenytoin.

complaints and Table 5.2 lists the common endocrine disorders that may present themselves to you in clinical practice, alongside a cluster of associated signs and symptoms.

Background History for the Endocrine System

Several medical conditions affecting the Endocrine system can run in families and a large number of dietary and environmental factors can play a part, so before you get started it's useful to establish the following [3, 4].

Table 5.2 Summary table of common Endocrine conditions and associated symptoms [2]

Common endocrine conditions	Common symptoms
Addison's Disease	Fatigue, anorexia, myalgia, low mood, weight loss, skin discolouration, polyuria.
Hypothyroidism	Fatigue, lethargy, weakness, weight gain, hoarse voice, goitre, dry skin, puffy face, oedema, constipation, cold intolerance, coarse hair and skin.
Hyperthyroidism	Excitability, anxiety, palpitations, heat intolerance, diarrhoea, weight loss, increased hair fall, goitre, fatigue and weakness / exhaustion, gritty eyes, eye swelling, diplopia.
Infertility	Irregular or absent menstruation, weight gain, reduced libido, vaginal dryness, pelvic pain.
Diabetes mellitus	Polyuria, polydipsia, blurred vision, weight loss, polyphagia, fatigue, lethargy, parasthesiae, repeated infections, thrush, poor wound healing.
Polycystic ovarian syndrome (PCOS)	Irregular or absent menstruation, hirsutism, androgenic alopecia, acne, greasy skin.
Hypogonadism	Irregular or absent menstruation (females), erectile dysfunction (males), low libido, infertility, fatigue, low mood, loss of secondary sexual characteristics e.g. reduced shaving frequency.
Hyperprolactinaemia	Galactorrhoea, headaches, bitemporal hemianopia, absent or irregular menstruation, low libido, erectile dysfunction, gynaecomastia.
Cushing's syndrome	Weight gain, skin thinning, easy bruising, moon face, buffalo hump, centripetal weight gain, mood disturbances, striae, acne, slow wound healing, low libido, infertility.
Hypopituitarism	Irregular or absent menstruation, loss of secondary sexual characteristics, fatigue, mood disturbances, reduced quality of life, features of other deficiencies e.g. hypothyroidism.
Acromegaly	Enlarged peripheries, enlarged skull bones and facial features, polyarthralgia, parasthesiae, glossomegaly, headaches, bitemporal hemianopia, widely spaced teeth, cardiomegaly, coarse, oily, thickened skin.

- History of previous medical or surgical problems and any previous investigations such as neurosurgery, renal operations or radiotherapy?
- Do they have a family history of any Endocrine conditions (especially Diabetes, thyroid disorders and neuro-endocrine cancers as these can have a genetic component)?
- Medications—multiple drugs, both prescribed, for example anti-psychotics and anti-coagulants, and recreational e.g. cannabis, anabolic steroids bought doen the gym, as well as alcohol can impact the endocrine system. Make sure that you get a full list of what they are taking.
- Constitutional upset—have they lost any weight recently? Have their diet or eating patterns changed?
- Menstrual history—this is very relevant to Endocrine conditions such as PCOS and thyroid and pituitary disorders, but also diabetes and more.

GOITRE = an enlargement of the thyroid gland [5]

Onset + Duration
- When did you first notice the swelling in your neck?
- Did the swelling increase in size slowly or rapidly?

Establishing the time frame helps to rationalise as to whether this is an acute inflammatory type process e.g. thyroiditis, or a chronic, insidious enlargement as one might find in Hashimoto's.

Discomfort
- Do you have any pain or tenderness over the area of swelling in your neck?

An acutely swollen thyroid gland can be uncomfortable and tender to the touch.

Pressure Symptoms
- Have you noticed difficulty swallowing, or do you feel like there is a lump in your throat?
- Do you have any difficulty breathing or shortness of breath?
- Do you have a hoarse voice or any voice changes?

It is important to understand the extent of potential compromise to surrounding structures and these questions will help to identify as to whether additional investigations are required such as swallowing tests e.g. barium studies, laryngoscopy to examine the vocal folds, or spirometry to assess airflow.

Thyroid Hormone Disturbance

See section below. Goitre can present with hypothyroidism, euthyroidism or hyperthyroidism.

Medication
- Are you taking any medication that might affect your thyroid function?
- Have you ever taken thyroid hormone replacement therapy?

For example, amiodarone, lithium, or iodine-containing supplements, are all 'goitrogens'.

Environment
- Have you ever lived in or visited an area of Iodine deficiency?
- Have you had any radiation exposure to the head or neck area?

Certain parts of the world have endemic low levels of iodine leading to 'Derbyshire Neck'.

Common Causes of Goitre [6]

Environmental	Iodine deficiency is more common in remote inland areas; South-East Asia, China, India, Nepal, Kazakhstan, Derbyshire
	Substances found in certain foods (e.g., cruciferous vegetables like cabbage or cassava) can interfere with thyroid hormone production, leading to goitre in regions where iodine deficiency is prevalent.
Endocrine	Hypothyroidism, Hashimoto's thyroiditis, Grave's disease
	Thyroid nodular disease, Thyroid Cancer, Thyroid cystic disease
	TSHoma.
Physiological	Pregnancy, menopause.
Auto-immune	De Quervain's Thyroiditis.
Medications	Lithium, Amiodrone, Iodine excess
Infiltration	Tuberculosis, Sarcoidosis

Approach to Management

Each of these causes requires careful evaluation through medical history, diagnostic tests, and imaging to guide appropriate treatment [5]. Neck examination is useful to assess whether the goitre feels tender, hard ('woody') or lumpy. Assessing whether the goitre moves on swallowing helps identify whether it is attached to surrounding structures. Don't forget to look for features of hypo and hyper-thyroidism and also examine the eyes for features of thyroid eye disease such as lid lag and diplopia.

Blood tests	FBC, U&E's, LFT's, T3, T4, TSH
	Thyroid auto-antibodies, anti-TPO, anti-TSH and TRAbs.
	Pituitary profile, 9 AM cortisol
	Inflammatory markers
Imaging	Thyroid ultrasound +/− FNAC if concerning nodules or lesions.
	Thyroid uptake scan with Iodine 131 if considering thyroiditis or unclear aetiology.
	CT or MRI neck if concerned about local mass effect
	Laryngoscopy / upper GI endoscopy if concerned about voice or swallowing
Other	Spirometry to assess air flow / degree of obstruction.
Treatment	Analgesia (avoid Aspirin) if painful
	Support airway if compromised or risk of aspiration
	Treat the underlying cause.
	Surgery if evidence of significant mass effect.
Red flags	Airway or voice compromise
	Exquisite tenderness (may indicate haemorrhage).

FATIGUE = Extreme tiredness / tired all the time [7]

Characterisation
- Can you describe what you mean by fatigue?

Getting a verbatim description 'feeling like death warmed up', 'I feel like wading through treacle' is useful, characterisations of fatigue means different things to different people.

Onset + Duration
- When did the fatigue start?
- Do you feel tired all the time or does it come and go?
- Was the onset sudden or gradual?

It is useful to get an idea of the time course of fatigue and understand whether it is acute or chronic.

Pattern + Progression
- Is the fatigue worsening, improving, or staying the same?
- Is there any relief with rest or sleep?

Does the fatigue relate to specific events and precipitants and recover from rest as one might expect, or is it all encompassing with no relief.

Severity + Impact
- How severe is the fatigue on a scale of 1–10?
- How is it affecting your daily activities (work, social life, etc.)?
- Are there specific times of day when it is worse?

You need to ascertain a quantifiable measure of the fatigue in order to understand its impact and track changes over time.

Sleep + Rest
- How many hours do you sleep each night?
- Do you feel refreshed when you wake up?
- Do you experience difficulty falling asleep, staying asleep, or waking early?
- Do you snore or has anyone noticed periods of stopped breathing during sleep?

Sleep quantity and quality are useful indicators.
If the individual is not getting high quality refreshing sleep then review their sleep hygiene and also ask about snoring (check with their partner) as they could have obstructive sleep apnoea.
Poor quality sleep and poor sleep habits are signs of depression.

Associated Symptoms
- Weight loss or gain?
- Fever or night sweats?
- Changes in your skin or hair?
- Changes in appetite or bowel habits?
- Muscle or joint pains?
- Depression, anxiety, or stress?

- Are you currently experiencing significant stress at work, home, or in relationships?
- Have there been any recent life changes, such as a new job, loss of a loved one, or financial stress?
- Have you been feeling down, hopeless, or disinterested in things that normally bring you joy?
- Memory or concentration issues?
- Any issues with headaches or dizziness?

Constitutional upset may reveal an underlying serious condition such as a chronic indolent infection or malignancy. It is important to identify any GI disorder leading to malabsorption and malnutrition.

Rheumatological disorders can lead to muscle inflammation, weakness and fatigue. Ask specifically about mental health and life events. Is there something keeping them up at night? Is there a background history of depression for instance? Consider neuro-psychological disorders as contributors to fatigue.

Medications + Alcohol
- Are you taking any sedatives?
- How much have you been drinking recently?

Review the medication list to look for treatments that may have an effect on energy levels.

Alcohol excess or changes in drinking patterns can lead to fatigue.

Exposure
- Have you had any recent infections, such as colds, flu, or COVID-19?
- Have you travelled recently, especially to areas where certain infections (e.g. malaria) are prevalent?

Post-viral fatigue is a recognised phenomenon so ask about the prodrome of the fatigue and occurrence of recent illnesses. Foreign travel may provide a clue as to a potential communicable disease that could be implicated in fatigue.

Common Causes of Fatigue [8]

Endocrine	Newly diagnosed or poorly controlled Diabetes mellitus
	Hypothyroidism, Adreno-cortical insufficiency, Cushing's syndrome
	Menopause, hypogonadism
Haematological	Anaemia, chronic bleeding, leukaemia, lymphoma.
Cardiac	Congestive cardiac failure, coronary artery disease / myocardial insufficiency, arrhythmias.
Respiratory	Obstructive sleep apnoea, Asthma, COPD.
GI	Malabsorption e.g. coeliac disease, IBD, pernicious anaemia,
	Chronic liver disease

(continued)

Neurological	Cerebrovascular disease, multiple sclerosis, Parkinson's disease, chronic fatigue syndrome.
Musculo-skeletal	Chronic pain syndromes, fibromyalgia, rheumatoid arthritis, SLE.
Psychiatric	Anxiety, stress, depression, burnout.
Infectious disease	Fatigue is common during and after infections due to immune response
	Viral infections (e.g. mononucleosis, COVID-19, flu).
	Chronic infections (e.g. Tuberculosis, HIV/AIDS).
	Persistent infections can cause ongoing fatigue.
	Post-viral fatigue. Fatigue may persist even after recovery from the initial viral illness.
Metabolic	Chronic renal disease and uraemia
	Electrolyte imbalance e.g. hyponatraemia and hypokalaemia
	Vitamin deficiencies e.g. B12, iron, folate, vitamin D.
	Obesity—due to the additional effort required for ADL's
Medications	Sedatives, antihistamines, beta-blockers, and certain antidepressants can cause fatigue as a side effect.
Malignancy	Both cancer itself and its treatments (chemotherapy, radiation) can cause profound fatigue.

Approach to Management

The causes of fatigue span multiple systems and require a detailed history, examination, and investigations to identify the underlying issue [9].

Blood tests	FBC, U&E's, LFT'S, TFT's
	Serum electrolytes including calcium and magnesium
	Inflammatory markers
	Haematinics / blood film / Fe studies
	Vitamin D
	9 AM Cortisol, 9 AM Testosterone (if indicated)
	Fasting blood glucose / random glucose / HbA1c
	Viral serology (e.g. Epstein-Barr virus, HIV, Hepatitis panel)
	Auto-immune screening (e.g. ANA, ANCA, Rheumatoid factor)
Imaging	CXR
	Echocardiography (if indicated)
Other	ECG
	Epworth sleepiness scale score
	Sleep studies (polysomnography)
	Psychological screening tools (e.g. PHQ-9, GAD-7)

(continued)

Treatment	Emphasise good sleep hygiene and routine
	Maintain good diet, nutrition and hydration
	Reduce or eliminate alcohol
	Relaxation techniques and self-care
	Treat the underlying abnormality
Red flags	Daytime somnolence
	Significant weight loss
	Night sweats

GALACTORRHOEA = spontaneous flow of milk or a milk-like secretion from the breast(s), unrelated to childbirth or breastfeeding [10]

Character
- Can you describe the type of discharge that you are getting?
- What is the colour of the discharge (e.g. milky, clear, bloody, yellow)?
- Is the discharge from one or both breasts?
- How much discharge is present (e.g. drops vs. more significant amounts)?

The type, quantity and site (one or both) of the breast discharge will provide information about the potential underlying cause. If thick and discoloured, then infection is likely. If bloody, suggests trauma of significant underlying breast pathology. Plentiful, free flowing 'milky' discharge is more likely related to prolactin disorders.

Onset + Duration
- When did you first notice the nipple discharge?
- Is the discharge persistent or intermittent?
- Did the discharge start suddenly or gradually?

Understand whether this is gradual or rapidly progressive. Does it happen all the time or was there an identifiable trigger?

Precipitants
- Is the discharge spontaneous, or does it occur only with nipple stimulation or pressure?
- Any recent chest wall trauma?
- Have you noticed any skin changes, especially around the breasts or armpits?
- Do you regularly engage in activities that involve breast or nipple stimulation?
- Do you think that you might be pregnant?
- Have you been pregnant or breastfed recently?

Can the patient identify anything specific that stimulates the breast tissue and as such acts as a reinforcing cycle for milk production. If the patient has had unprotected sex recently then it makes sense to undertake a pregnancy test even if they have been using contraception.

Associations
- Have you noticed any breast pain, tenderness, or lumps?
- Any changes in breast size?
- Have you experienced any changes in your menstrual cycle (e.g. irregular periods, missed periods)?
- Do you have symptoms of polycystic ovary syndrome (PCOS), such as excess hair growth, acne, or irregular periods?
- Do you have headaches, vision problems, or difficulty seeing objects on the sides of your field of vision?

- Are you experiencing any symptoms of an underactive thyroid (e.g. weight gain, cold intolerance, fatigue)?
- Have you experienced any decreased libido or changes in sexual function?
- Have you had any difficulty getting pregnant?
- Have you noticed any changes in weight or energy levels?

Assess for potential direct breast pathology. Breasts can enlarge with pregnancy. Hormonal imbalances that cause galactorrhoea can also disrupt menstruation.

Focal neurological features suggest a pituitary issue with mass effect.

Ask about thyroid symptoms, hypothyroidism causes increased precursors such as TRH to be produced, this also stimulates Prolactin production.

Low libido and infertility are clues to hypogonadism in both males and females. Infertility suggests a chronic underlying hormonal imbalance.

Weight loss will make you consider constitutional upset and look for evidence of other significant pathology.

Medications
- Birth control pills or hormone replacement therapy?
- Antipsychotic or antidepressant medications (e.g. risperidone, haloperidol)?
- Blood pressure medications (e.g. verapamil)?
- Gastrointestinal drugs (e.g. metoclopramide)?
- Do you use recreational drugs (e.g. marijuana, opioids)?
- Are you taking any herbal supplements or over-the-counter drugs?

Multiple medications, drugs and supplements can precipitate galactorrhoea, largely through interference with dopamine neurotransmission.

Common Causes of Galactorrhoea [11]

Endocrine	Hyperprolactinaemia, prolactinoma.
	Co-secreting pituitary tumours (Acromegaly, Cushing's)
	Hypothyroidism, PCOS.
Neurological	Pituitary stalk compression / brain trauma.
Breast	Excessive manual stimulation, chest wall trauma or surgery, mammary duct ectasia.
Infiltration	Sarcoidosis, Tuberculosis.
Medications	Antipsychotics (e.g. risperidone, haloperidol)
	Antidepressants (e.g. SSRIs, tricyclics)
	Antihypertensives (e.g. methyldopa, verapamil)
	Prokinetics (e.g. metoclopramide)
	Oral contraceptives (hormonal influence on prolactin)
	Opioids
Metabolic	Chronic renal disease, liver cirrhosis
Psychiatric	Severe emotional and physical stress (prolactin is a 'stress hormone')

Approach to Management

These questions and a thorough examination will help assess potential causes of galactorrhoea, including hormonal imbalances (e.g. hyperprolactinemia), medication side effects, thyroid dysfunction, or underlying breast pathology [10].

Blood tests	FBC, U&E's, LFT's, TFT's
	Anterior pituitary profile (Prolactin, LH, FSH, IGF-1, 9 AM cortisol, testosterone/ oestradiol depending on gender)
	Inflammatory markers.
	Cannulated prolactin (if borderline result / suggestion of stress)
Imaging	MRI Pituitary (once biochemical diagnosis confirmed)
	Breast ultrasound / mammography (if indicated)
Treatment	Reduce breast manipulation
	Breast pads
	Treat the underlying cause
	Withdraw / replace offending medications if possible
	May require Dopamine agonists if hyperprolactinaemia
Red flags	Evidence of local pituitary mass effects—request early neurosurgical assessment.
	Presence of breast lumps—refer to breast team for urgent review.

GYNAECOMASTIA = presence of excessive breast tissue (males). It is characterised by the presence of palpable, firm, glandular tissue beneath the nipple, as opposed to the fatty tissue found in obesity (pseudogynaecomastia) [12]

Onset + Duration
- When did you first notice the breast enlargement?
- Has the enlargement been gradual or sudden?
- Is the enlargement in one or both breasts?
- Has the size of the breast tissue changed over time?

The time course of the breast tissue enlargement will help identify the underlying pathology.

Associations
- Do you experience any pain, tenderness, or discomfort in the breast area?
- Have you noticed any nipple discharge (e.g. clear, milky, or bloody)?
- Do you feel any lumps or have you noticed changes in the skin or nipple?
- Do you have any changes in sexual function, such as reduced libido, erectile dysfunction, or changes in testicular size?

It is important to explore whether this is primary breast pathology. These questions also relate to the potential presence of hypogonadism.

Puberty and Development
- Did you have normal development during puberty?
- Have you ever had breast enlargement during adolescence, and did it resolve?

Medications
- Have you recently stopped or started any new medications?
- Are you taking any of the following;
- Hormonal treatments (e.g. testosterone therapy, anabolic steroids)
- Antipsychotics (e.g. risperidone, haloperidol)
- Antidepressants (e.g. SSRIs, tricyclics)
- Antiandrogens (e.g. spironolactone, finasteride, flutamide)
- Prostate cancer treatments (e.g. bicalutamide, oestrogen therapy)
- Cardiac medications (e.g. digoxin, calcium channel blockers, amiodarone)
- Antiulcer medications (e.g. cimetidine, omeprazole)
- Chemotherapy drugs

A variety of medications can interfere with the endocrine system and can cause alterations in relative testosterone and oestrogen levels precipitating breast tissue development.

Drugs + Alcohol
- How much alcohol do you consume, and how often?
- Do you engage in bodybuilding or take any supplements (e.g. protein powders, over-the-counter hormones)?
- Do you take any recreational drugs (e.g. marijuana, alcohol, heroin)?

Narcotics and supplements can interfere with hormonal regulation, especially horse steroids purchased at the gym.

Endocrine Dysfunction
- Have you noticed changes in hair growth (e.g. loss of body hair)?
- Do you have changes in muscle mass or feel generally weaker than before?
- Have you experienced hot flushes or mood changes?
- Do you have any problems with your erections such as loss of spontaneous morning erections?
- Have you had any issues with infertility?

These are all features of hypogonadism, or the 'andropause' in men.

Associated Conditions
- Do you have any known hormonal disorders, such as hypogonadism (low testosterone) or hyperthyroidism?
- Have you ever been diagnosed with liver disease, kidney disease, or a thyroid disorder?
- Do you have any history of testicular injury, surgery, or infection (e.g. mumps orchitis)?
- Have you experienced any significant weight loss or gain recently?
- Do you have a family history of breast cancer or testicular cancer?

Pre-existing medical conditions can interfere with hormone metabolism and give rise to oestrogen dominance.

Common Causes of Gynaecomastia [13]

Endocrine	Hypogonadism, Klinefelter's syndrome, Primary testicular failure
	Hyperthyroidism (raises levels of SHBG and increases free oestrogen)
	Adrenal tumours secreting oestrogen
	Androgen insensitivity syndrome (unopposed oestrogen action)
	Testicular trauma, infection, tumours
	Pituitary tumours, hyperprolactinaemia
Metabolic	Liver disease e.g. cirrhosis, alcohol excess, chronic kidney disease
Medications	Spironolactone, finasteride, bicalutamide (anti-androgens)
	Cimetidine, Ketoconazole, PPI's
	Anti-psychotics, anti-depressants, Benzodiazepines
	Anabolic steroids
Physiological	Pubertal gynaecomastia (transient imbalance between oestrogen and testosterone).

Approach to Management

The assessment for gynaecomastia focuses on identifying potential causes such as medications, hormonal imbalances, systemic illnesses, and lifestyle factors (e.g. drug use, alcohol). Detailed exploration of the patient's reproductive health, symptoms, and underlying conditions can help in diagnosing the cause of gynaecomastia using a holistic approach. Examine secondary sexual characteristics and look for evidence of other systemic illness e.g. liver disease [12, 13].

Blood tests	FBC, U&Es, LFT's, TFT's
	Anterior pituitary profile (Prolactin, LH, FSH, IGF-1, 9 AM cortisol, 9 AM testosterone, 17 beta Oestradiol, SHBG), hCG.
Imaging	Breast ultrasound / mammography (if indicated)
	MRI Pituitary (if indicated)
	Testicular ultrasound (if indicated)
	Adrenal phase CT (if indicated)
Treatment	Withdraw any offending agents
	Treat the underlying cause
	Reduction mammoplasty surgery (if unresolved or problematic)
	Anti-oestrogenic medication e.g. Tamoxifen, Clomiphene
Red flags	Abnormal breast lumps (breast cancer is rare in men)
	Testicular lumps
	Pituitary mass effects

MENSTRUAL DISTURBANCE = an irregularity of menstruation in terms of intensity, duration, timing or complete cessation [14]

Menarche/Cycle
- How old were you when you originally started having periods?
- Did you go through a normal puberty as far as you know?
- What is the normal frequency and pattern of your periods?
- How many days is your typical menstrual cycle (from the start of one period to the start of the next)?

Clarifying at what age the individual first started menstruating is useful—as well as making sure that they did in fact experience menarche (primary vs secondary amenorrhoea)—also understand what their normal menstrual cycle is like so that you can evaluate the delta.

Onset + Duration
- When was your last menstrual period (LMP)?
- When did you notice a change in your periods?
- Was this a gradual change e.g. interval gradually getting longer or shorter?
- Have you experienced any extended periods of time without menstruation?

The time course of change can sometimes be difficult to discern, although many women now use period tracking apps which are a useful source of data.

Characteristics
- How frequent are your periods now?
- How many days does your period last?
- How heavy is the flow (e.g. number of pads or tampons used per day, presence of clots)?
- Have you noticed any changes in the heaviness of your flow over time?

Getting periods every 21 days or less is known as **polymenorrhoea**, more than every 35 days is **oligomenorrhea** (less than 9 periods in 12 months). Complete cessation of periods after a previously normal history of menstruation is known as secondary amenorrhoea.

- Do you have any bleeding between periods (intermenstrual bleeding)?
- Do you experience bleeding after intercourse (postcoital bleeding)?

These symptoms may indicate uterine, cervical or vaginal pathology.

Associated Symptoms
- Do you experience pain during your periods?
- Is the pain mild, moderate, or severe?
- Does it interfere with your daily activities?
- When does the pain start (before, during, or after menstruation)?

- Do you experience pelvic pain at other times during the cycle (e.g. mid-cycle pain)?

Painful periods are known as dysmenorrhea and occur on a spectrum of severity.

- Do you experience premenstrual symptoms such as bloating, breast tenderness, mood swings, or irritability?
- Have you had any hot flushes, night sweats, or vaginal dryness (suggestive of perimenopause or menopause)?

Again, gauge what is normal and what has changed for the patient. Symptoms of oestrogen withdrawal such as with the menopause or primary ovarian insufficiency can be very pronounced.

- Do you think that you could be pregnant?

Unprotected intercourse—do a pregnancy test.

Other Medical Conditions
- Do you have any known hormonal or endocrine disorders (e.g. PCOS, hypothyroidism, hyperthyroidism, diabetes)?
Hormonal imbalances from other systems can disrupt the menstrual cycle.

- Have you had any previous gynaecological surgeries?

For example, fibroid removal, endometriosis treatment, hysterectomy.

- Is there a family history of menstrual irregularities, early menopause, PCOS, or gynaecological cancers?

Menopausal age tends to run in families so it's worth asking if the patient knows when their mother went through the menopause.

- Do you have any chronic medical conditions?
- Are you currently taking any medications, including hormonal treatments, birth control pills, or herbal supplements?
- Have you recently started or stopped any medications (e.g. antidepressants, anti-coagulants, steroids)?

Liver disease, kidney disease, chronic infections, autoimmune conditions etc. can all interfere with menstruation.

Lifestyle
- Have you experienced significant weight changes (weight gain or loss) recently?
- Do you engage in intense physical exercise or have a history of eating disorders (e.g. anorexia, bulimia)?
- Are you under a lot of stress or anxiety?
- Have you been diagnosed with depression or other mental health conditions?
- Do you use alcohol, tobacco, or recreational drugs? If so, how frequently?

Hypothalamic amenorrhoea is a well-recognised phenomenon often occurring in young women who are under physical or emotional pressures.

Common Causes of Menstrual Disorders [15]

Endocrine	Thyroid disease, hyperprolactinaemia, hypogonadism / POI, Cushing's.
	Delayed puberty (if primary amenorrhoea after age 15)
Gynaecological	PCOS, Endometriosis, Uterine fibroids / polyps, PID
Metabolic	Chronic illness e.g. CKD, liver disease. Alcohol excess.
Medication	Contraceptive medication, antidepressants, antipsychotics, anticoagulants, steroids.
Psychological	Stress, anxiety, depression, eating disorders
Physiological	Pregnancy, hypothalamic amenorrhoea, intense exercise, weight loss, malnutrition.
	Perimenopause / menopause

Approach to Management

A thorough medical history is essential to identify the underlying cause of menstrual disturbances. The history should focus on the pattern of menstruation, associated symptoms, medical conditions, lifestyle factors, and potential risk factors. This helps guide further diagnostic testing and management strategies [16]. BMI measurement is useful to record.

Blood tests	FBC, U&E's, LFT's, TFT's
	Anterior pituitary profile (Prolactin, LH, FSH, IGF-1, 9 AM cortisol, TSH)
	Androgen profile, 17 beta Oestradiol, 17OH Progesterone, SHBG.
	Beta HCG.
	Inflammatory markers
	Clotting profile
Imaging	Pelvic ultrasound
	Pituitary MRI (if indicated)
	Hysteroscopy (if indicated)
Treatment	Diary (or app) to record menstrual pattern
	Analgesia for pain
	Tamoxifen if menorrhagia
	Treat the underlying cause
	If oestrogen deficient consider HRT (for wellbeing and bone protection)
	Consider progesterone if prolonged time with no bleeding to stimulate shedding of the endometrial lining and overcome the effects of unopposed oestrogen.
Red flags	Intermenstrual bleeding
	Menorrhagia leading to anaemia
	Rapid virilisation (suggests adrenal tumour)
	Unexplained weight loss

HIRSUTISM = the development of male pattern excessive hair growth in a female [17].

Characterisation
- Can you describe the types of hair that you've been developing?
- Where exactly do you have excess hair (e.g. face, chest, abdomen, back)?
- How dense or thick is the hair in those areas?

Thick, dark, stubbly hair is more likely to be androgen driven, as opposed to thin, fairer longer hair types. The key here is to identify whether the hair growth is similar to a male-pattern hair distribution.

Onset + Duration
- When did you first notice the excessive hair growth?
- Has the hair growth been gradual or sudden?
- Has it worsened over time, or has it stayed the same?

This helps to establish the timeframe and potential underlying causes. It is also useful to establish what is normal for the individual. Asking for a photo of how they looked at baseline is a good guide.

Menstrual Disturbance
- See question set above.

Indicates a potential hormonal imbalance.

Features of Hyperandrogenism
Have you noticed any of the following;

- Acne or oily skin?
- Thinning hair on the scalp (male-pattern baldness)?
- Deepening of your voice?
- Increased muscle mass?

All of these are features suggestive of testosterone excess. Rapid virilisation (becoming more male) is a concerning feature of a potential malignancy.

Medications
- Are you currently taking any medications? (specifically ask about androgens, steroids, birth control pills, or other hormonal treatments)
- Are you using any over-the-counter supplements, herbal remedies, or anabolic steroids?

All of these agents can interfere with androgen metabolism.

Weight and Lifestyle
- Have you had any significant weight changes recently?
- Do you have difficulty losing or gaining weight?
- Do you exercise regularly or follow a specific diet?

Syndromes of insulin resistance such as PCOS are closely linked to excess weight. Weight loss is a useful non-medical management approach to improving hirsutism.

Endocrine Disorders
- Have you experienced any symptoms of type 2 diabetes such as excessive thirst, going to the toilet more frequently, blurring of your eyesight or loss of energy?

In the context of certain risk factors such as being overweight, signs and symptoms of the metabolic syndrome may be more common.

- Have you experienced any symptoms of thyroid dysfunction such as weight changes, intolerance to heat or cold, fatigue, or palpitations?

Both thyroid overactivity and underactivity can alter the balance of sex hormones and contribute to hirsutism.

- Have you had symptoms suggestive of Cushing's syndrome (e.g. weight gain, especially around the abdomen, purple stretch marks, easy bruising)?

Cushing's is a rare condition that can contribute to hirsutism but is often missed because it is not considered.

Family History
- Does anyone in your family (e.g., mother, sisters) have a history of hirsutism or excessive hair growth?
- Is there a family history of conditions such as **polycystic ovary syndrome (PCOS)**, **diabetes**, or **thyroid disorders**?

Useful to ascertain whether there is a combination of both environmental and genetic factors.

Hair Management
- What treatments have you tried for controlling the hair growth; shaving, waxing, plucking, laser?
- Did the treatment help in reducing the hair growth?

Mechanical methods of hair growth may work in the short term but if the underlying cause is not treated then male pattern hair growth, especially facial hair can worsen.

Common Causes of Hirsutism [18]

Endocrine	PCOS (if fulfilling the modified Rotterdam diagnostic criteria)
	Congenital adrenal hyperplasia (non-classical)
	Cushing's syndrome
	Thyroid disorders
	Adrenal tumours
	Insulin resistance syndromes / type 2 diabetes.
Gynaecological	Ovarian tumours (androgen secreting tumours can cause rapid virilisation), Theca cell hyperplasia (causing overproduction of androgens).
Physiological	Pregnancy (increased androgen production during pregnancy due to hormonal changes).
	Genetic / familial hirsutism—seen in multiple family members, particularly in women from certain ethnic groups (e.g. Mediterranean, Middle Eastern, South Asian descent).
Medication	Androgenic drugs including testosterone replacement therapy, spironolactone.
	Anabolic steroids, Glucocorticoids, Danazol, Minoxidil.

Approach to Management

Hirsutism, or excessive hair growth in women in areas where hair growth is typically minimal or absent, can result from various causes, often related to increased androgen production or sensitivity [18, 19].

Blood tests	FBC, U&E's, LFT's, TFT's
	Anterior pituitary profile (Prolactin, LH, FSH, IGF-1, 9 AM cortisol, TSH)
	Androgen profile, 17 beta Oestradiol, 17OH Progesterone, SHBG.
	Short synacthen test with progesterone levels (if indicated)
Imaging	Pituitary MRI (if indicated)
	Ovarian ultrasound (if indicated)
	CT adrenals (if indicated)
Other	Ferriman-Galway score (quantitative assessment of the extent of hirsutism)
Treatment	Weight loss guidance and dietician referral
	Manual hair removal techniques
	Consider trial of Eflornithine cream (Vaniqa) may take up to 6 months of persistent use to have an effect.
	Treat the underlying cause.
	If PCOS is diagnosed, Metformin is often used first line to reduce insulin resistance and support weight loss.
Red flags	Rapid pattern of development of male secondary sexual characteristics.

THYROID HORMONE DISORDERS = over or under activity of thyroid hormone can lead to symptoms of sluggish or excess metabolism respectively [20].

Onset + Duration
- How long have you been feeling unwell for?

Patients may be non-specifically unwell with vague, insidious symptoms and no clear inciting incident. Both over and under active thyroid disorders can evolve slowly. TSH has a half-life of several weeks. Thyroiditis can be acute due to inflammation and sudden release of preformed T4.

Energy Levels
- Have you experienced unusual fatigue, excessive tiredness, or the feeling of too much energy?
- How is your exercise tolerance?

People with hypothyroidism generally feel tired and sluggish.
In hyperthyroidism individuals may initially feel very energetic but can become exhausted.

Muscle Weakness
- Do you feel muscle weakness or tremors in your hands or legs?

Hypothyroidism leads to reductions in strength, endurance and myalgia.
Hyperthyroidism can lead to twitches, spasms and tremors.

Weight Changes
- Have you noticed any unexpected weight gain or weight loss?

Classic signs of abnormal metabolic activity. These changes normally happen outwith any diet or activity changes.

Temperature Intolerance
- Do you feel excessively cold or hot compared to others?

Another classic sign, often picked up in relation to close contacts.

Skin and Hair
- Have you noticed any changes in your skin (dryness, paleness) or hair (thinning, loss)?

Hypothyroidism leads to coarse, dry skin and hair. Hyperthyroidism may lead to increased hair fall.

Change in Bowel Habit
- Have you had any changes in your bowel movements, such as constipation or diarrhoea?

Slow transit commonly occurs in hypothyroidism, whereas, rapid, frequent bowel motions are a sign of hyperthyroidism.

Mood Changes
- Have you experienced anxiety, depression, irritability, or changes in your emotional state?

Asking about the patient's mental health is an important gauge as hormones shape the way we think and feel. Hypothyroidism leads people to feel low in mood, blue and tearful. Hyperthyroidism can lead to anxiety and stress, plus irritability.

Menstrual Disturbance
- Have you noticed changes in your menstrual cycle (irregular, heavier, or lighter periods)?

Thyroid disorders can lead to hormone imbalance, stress on the metabolism and interference with menses.

Palpitations
- Have you experienced palpitations, irregular heartbeats, or a noticeable change in heart rate?

Hypothyroidism slows the heart rate and predisposes to bradycardia and heart failure.
Hyperthyroidism can lead to palpitations, tachycardia and arrhythmias.

Neck Problems
- Have you felt any swelling, tightness, or discomfort in your neck?
- Have you noticed any changes in your voice or difficulty swallowing?

Development of a goitre, or inflammation and pain with thyroiditis can present in tandem with metabolic disturbances.

Eye Signs
- Have you noticed any problems with your eyes recently?
  Ask about change in appearance/swelling, double vision, grittiness, irritability.
Thyroid eye disease is inflammatory and important to pick up.

Sleep Quality
- Have you had trouble sleeping or experienced insomnia?

Thyroid disorders can lead to interference with high quality, refreshing sleep.

Diet
- Do you consume a diet high or low in iodine (e.g. iodized salt, seafood, or seaweed)?

Several dietary factors have been shown to interfere with thyroid hormone levels. Has the patient been to an area of endemically low iodine (see goitre section).

Family History
- Does anyone in your family have a history of thyroid disorders (hypothyroidism, hyperthyroidism, thyroid cancer)?

Thyroid disorders tend to run in families, often through the female line.
Also ask about other auto-immune conditions.

Medical History

- Do you have a history of autoimmune disorders (e.g. lupus, rheumatoid arthritis, type 1 diabetes)?

The presence of 1 auto-immune condition increases the risks of others developing.

- Have you had any surgery or radiation therapy to your neck?
- Are you on any medications that might affect thyroid function, such as lithium, amiodarone, or corticosteroids?

Predisposing factors to thyroid irritation.

- Have you used iodine-containing supplements or medications (e.g. contrast agents for imaging studies)?

Drugs that interfere with iodine can precipitate thyroid hormone disturbances.

Common Causes of Thyroid Disorders [21]

Endocrine	Hypothalamic-pituitary disorders e.g. hypopituitarism, TSHoma
Autoimmune	Hashimoto's thyroiditis, Grave's disease, Postpartum thyroiditis
Infection	De Quervain's subacute thyroiditis
Environmental	Iodine deficiency, iodine excess, radiation exposure, selenium deficiency
Medication	Amiodarone, Lithium, anti-thyroid medication e.g. Carbimazole
Genetic	Thyroid hormone resistance
Traumatic	Neck surgery or trauma

Approach to Management

These questions will help guide further diagnostic testing and physical examination to assess thyroid function and determine the presence of disorders like hypothyroidism, hyperthyroidism, or thyroid structural abnormalities (e.g. nodules or goitre) [22, 23]. Don't forget to examine for signs of thyroid eye disease.

Blood tests	FBC, U&E's, LFT's, T3, T4, TSH
	Thyroid auto-antibodies, anti-TPO, anti-TSH and TRAbs.
	Pituitary profile, 9 AM Cortisol
	Inflammatory markers
Imaging	Thyroid ultrasound if nodules or goitre
	Radionuclide thyroid scan (if indicated)
	Pituitary MRI scan (if indicated)
	Cardiac ECHO (if signs suggestive of cardiac failure)
	DEXA bone scan (to assess bone mineral density)
Treatment	Supportive measures depending on thyroid under or over activity
	Passive warming, hydration
	Propranolol for symptoms of thyrotoxicosis
	Anti-thyroid medication for hyperthyroidism
	Levo-thyroxine replacement therapy for hypothyroidism
	Treat the underlying cause where possible.
Red flags	Reduced conscious level (be wary of myxoedma coma)
	Congestive or high output cardiac failure
	Features of thyroid eye disease esp. diplopia or oculo-motor nerve palsies.

ERECTILE DYSFUNCTION = sub-optimal erectile function in males leading often leading to problems with penetrative sex [24]

Characterisation
- Have you been having any problems getting an erection recently?
- Can you describe a bit more about what you mean by this?
- Are you still getting spontaneous erections first thing in the morning when you wake up?

What does the individual mean by erectile dysfunction. Erections tend to be less satisfactory from middle age onwards.

Spontaneous morning erections are a good marker of testosterone status as levels of this hormone tend to peak first thing in the day.

Onset + Duration
- When did you first notice problems with getting or maintaining an erection?
- Was the onset sudden or gradual?
- Has the problem been continuous or does it occur intermittently?

Clarifying the time course is useful as this can tie to the underlying pathology.

Severity and Intensity
- How often do you experience difficulty with erections?
- Is the problem affecting your ability to achieve an erection, maintain it, or both?
- Can you achieve an erection during masturbation or sleep (e.g. nightime or morning erections)?
- How would you rate your ability to maintain an erection for sexual intercourse (on a scale of 1–10)?

It's important to establish under what conditions the ED occurs. Severity ratings provide a baseline for purposes of comparison and the impacts of any treatments.

Libido
- Has there been any change in your sexual desire (libido)?
- Do you still feel aroused, but find it difficult to achieve an erection?
- Does the issue with erections occur with different partners or in different situations?

Libido is linked to mood, situation, environmental and partner cues as well as hormonal status.

Psychological Factors
- Are there any stressors in your relationship that might affect your sexual performance?
- Are you experiencing anxiety, depression, or stress that might be affecting your sexual function?

- Have you had any recent life events (e.g. job loss, death of a loved one) that might be impacting your mental well-being?
- Have you experienced performance anxiety or fear of failure during sexual activity?
- Do you get any problems with premature ejaculation?

Getting and maintaining an erection requires significant psychological input and there can be many interfering factors.

Hypogonadism

- Have you noticed any weight gain around your middle recently?
- Has there been any reduction in muscle mass?
- Have you noticed if you've been shaving less frequently recently?
- Have you noticed any changes in the size of your genitals recently?
- Any change in your body hair or changes in your voice?

Make sure to ask specifically about features of low testosterone that could coincide with the development of the ED.

Medical Conditions

- Do you have any chronic medical conditions such as diabetes, hypertension, heart disease, or kidney disease?
- Have you been diagnosed with any vascular conditions (e.g. atherosclerosis) or neurological disorders?
- Have you experienced any chest pain, shortness of breath, or other symptoms suggestive of heart disease?

Chronic medical conditions can affect the production and metabolism of testosterone.
Vascular conditions can affect penile blood supply.

- Have you had any pelvic or urological surgery, radiation treatment or pelvic trauma?

Consider iatrogenic damage to the penile nerve supply.

Medications

- Are you taking any medications that might affect sexual function, such as:
- **Antidepressants** (e.g. SSRIs, tricyclics)?
- **Blood pressure medications** (e.g. beta-blockers, diuretics)?
- **Hormonal treatments** (e.g. testosterone or oestrogen therapy)?
- **Anti-androgens** (e.g. medications for prostate cancer)?
- Do you use tobacco, alcohol, or recreational drugs (e.g. marijuana, cocaine)? How often?
- Have you recently started or stopped any medications that may be affecting your erections?

Many medications and narcotics can interfere with erectile function.

ED Rx

- Have you tried any treatments for erectile dysfunction before (e.g. oral medications like Viagra or Cialis, vacuum devices, injections)?
- If so, did they work, and did you experience any side effects?

Response to medications such as PDE5 inhibitors is a useful way of identifying if there is damage to the underlying erectile mechanism.

Common Causes of Erectile Dysfunction [25]

Endocrine	Hypogonadism, hypopituitarism, hyperprolactinaemia, thyroid dysfunction, diabetes
Vascular	Atherosclerosis, hypertension, peripheral vascular disease
Neurological	Neuropathy, Spinal cord injuries, Multiple sclerosis, Parkinson's
Medication	Anti-androgens e.g. Finasteride, Spironolactone.
	Anti-hypertensives e.g. beta blockers
	Anti-depressants e.g. SSRI's
Narcotics	Alcohol, cannabis, opioids, cocaine, tobacco.
Trauma	Surgery, physical trauma, prolonged cycle riding.
Psychological	Stress, anxiety, depression, relationship issues.

Approach to Management

Getting and maintaining an erection is a complex physiological process that requires adequate blood supply, intact nervous system signalling, appropriate levels of testosterone and psychological harmony. If anything interferes with these delicate processes then ED may be the consequence. Examination is important to characterise the level of secondary sexual characteristics, size of genitals and gonads (using an orchidometer), as well undertaking a prostate examination and paying attention to the cardiovascular system [26]. ED tends to precede IHD by approximately 5 years [27].

Blood tests	FBC, U&E's, LFT'S, TFT's
	9 AM Androgen profile including gonadotrophins
	Pituitary profile
	Inflammatory markers
	Lipid profile
	PSA (if indicated)
Imaging	Pituitary MRI (if indicated)
	Testicular ultrasound (if indicated)
Treatment	Treat the underlying cause where possible
	Trial of PDE5 inhibitors (if no contraindications)
	Mechanical devices e.g. vacuum pumps
	Pscyho-sexual counselling
Red flags	Testicular lumps
	Pituitary mass effects

POLYDIPSIA & POLYURIA = Polydipsia refers to excessive thirst and an increased intake of fluids. Polyuria is excessive urine production, typically defined as urine output greater than 3 litres per day in adults [28]

Quantification/Characterisation
- How often do you urinate during the day?
- How many times at night (nocturia)?
- Approximately how much urine do you pass each time?
- Has the amount noticeably increased?
- Is the urine clear, light, or dark in colour?
- How much water or other fluids do you drink each day?
- How many caffeinated drinks do you drink?
- Do you feel thirsty all the time, or is it worse at certain times of day (e.g. morning, evening)?
- Does drinking fluids reduce your thirst, or do you still feel thirsty after drinking?
- Do you feel dehydrated despite drinking a lot of water?

Onset + Duration
- When did you first notice an increase in your urination or thirst?
- Has the onset been sudden or gradual?
- Is this a constant issue or does it come and go?

Associated Symptoms
Have you noticed any other symptoms, such as:

- Unexplained weight loss or gain?
- Fatigue or weakness?
- Blurred vision?
- Dry mouth or dry skin?
- Muscle cramps or weakness?
- Increased hunger (polyphagia)?

It's helpful to gather further details about symptoms that an individual may be experiencing due to hyperosmolarity. Ask about any swelling in the legs, hands, or face, as these are all features of fluid overload.

Medical History
Have you been diagnosed with any conditions that might explain these symptoms, such as:

- **Diabetes mellitus**?
- **Diabetes insipidus**?
- **Kidney disease**?

- **Hypercalcaemia** or **hypokalaemia**?
- **Hyperthyroidism** or other hormonal disorders?

Glucose and electrolyte imbalances can activate the body's normal mechanisms for correcting any pertubations.

- Have you experienced recent infections, such as urinary tract infections (UTIs)?
- Do you experience any urgency, burning, or pain when urinating (dysuria)?
- Have you noticed blood in your urine or other changes in urine colour or smell?
- Do you have any known prostate problems (males)?

It is important to establish if there are other lower urinary tract symptoms that could be causing the problems.

- Have you been diagnosed with any psychiatric conditions?

Primary (psychogenic) polydipsia can be more common in those with mental health issues.

Medications
- Are you taking any medications that may affect your urination or thirst, such as:
- Diuretics (water pills)?
- Antipsychotics?
- Lithium (for bipolar disorder)?
- Corticosteroids?
- Have you recently started or stopped any medications?
- Do you consume alcohol or caffeine, and how much per day?

Diet and Lifestyle
- Have there been any changes in your diet, such as increased salt or sugar intake?
- How much physical activity do you engage in, and has your activity level changed recently?
- Do you live in a hot climate or engage in activities that cause excessive sweating?
- Have you been under any increased stress or emotional strain recently?
- Have you noticed any patterns in your behaviour, such as drinking excessive water out of habit (compulsive drinking)?

Family History
- Is there a family history of diabetes (Type 1 or Type 2), kidney disease, or other endocrine disorders?
- Do any close relatives have conditions related to excessive urination or thirst?

Common Causes of Polydipsia and Polyuria [29]

Endocrine	Diabetes mellitus, HHS, DKA
	Diabetes insipidus
	Hyperthyroidism
	Primary hyperaldosteronism (Conn's syndrome)
Renal	Chronic kidney disease (leads to reducing concentrating ability)
	Acute kidney injury (excess urine excretion in the recovery phase)
	Post obstructive diuresis e.g. following catheter removal
	Tubulo-interstitial nephritis, UTI's, cystitis
Psychological	Primary / psychogenic polydipsia, stress, excess fluid intake
Metabolic	Hypercalcaemia, hypokalaemia, pregnancy
Medication	Diuretics, Steroids, Lithium, SGLT-2 inhibitors, alcohol, caffeine.

Approach to Management

Both polyuria and polydipsia are hallmark hyperosmolar symptoms of diabetes but can also occur in other disorders that affect the body's fluid and electrolyte balance, urological disorders, and medication side effects. Quantification is important, as is establishing behaviours and habits around fluid intake [30].

Blood tests	FBC, U&E's, LFT's, TFT's
	Fasting plasma glucose, HbA1c, Ketones
	Calcium, Magnesium, PTH, Vitamin D
	Pituitary profile
	Renin:aldosterone ratio
	Arterial blood gas (if indicated)
Urine tests	Urinalysis, volume measurement
	Glucose, nitrites, white cell count, protein, ketones
	24 h urinary collection (Ca, K, Mg, Cl etc)
	Calcium: Creatinine ratio.
Imaging	Renal tract ultrasound (if indicated)
Treatment	Correct any underlying glucose or electrolyte abnormality
	Rehydration if fluid depleted
	Treat the underlying cause
Red flags	Significant weight loss, hyperglycaemia, ketonuria, acidosis.

GLUCOSE DISTURBANCES = normally the body maintains tight control of plasma blood glucose levels, hypoglycaemia (low blood glucose) and hyperglycaemia (high blood glucose) indicate loss of metabolic control or significant stressors from intercurrent illness or interfering factors [31]

Onset + Duration
- How long have you been getting abnormal glucose levels?
- Are your glucose levels usually high (hyperglycaemia), low (hypoglycaemia), or both?
- Is this a new or ongoing issue?
- Are your symptoms more frequent at certain times of day (e.g. mornings, after meals, during exercise)?
- Have you had any previous episodes of high or low blood glucose levels?

The patient may not know the details as fluctuations in glucose can often be asymptomatic.

Hypoglycaemia Symptoms
Do you ever feel:

- Shaky or nervous?
- Sweaty or clammy?
- Dizzy or light-headed?
- Hungry or nauseous?
- Confused or irritable?
- Experience palpitations or a fast heart rate?
- Loss of consciousness or seizures?

Features which reflect sub-optimal cerebral fuel supply are described as 'neuro-glycopenia'.

Hyperglycaemia Symptoms
Have you experienced symptoms such as:

- Increased thirst?
- Frequent urination?
- Unexplained weight loss?
- Fatigue or weakness?
- Blurred vision?
- Increased hunger?
- Dry mouth or skin?

These are all classic hyperosmolar symptoms of elevated glucose.

Diet
- Do you monitor your sugar or carbohydrate intake?
- Can you describe a typical day's meals and snacks?
- Do you follow any special diet (e.g. low-carb, keto, Mediterranean)?

It is useful to get a feel for the carbohydrate component of their regular diet.

- Do you consume alcohol? If so, how much and how often?

Alcohol action can lead to both high and low glucose readings at different time phases and also the type of alcohol (and mixers) consumed can have an influence.

Medications
- Are you taking any medications for blood sugar control (e.g. insulin, oral hypo-glycaemics like metformin, sulfonylureas)?
- Have you recently started or stopped any medications that might affect glucose levels (e.g. steroids, beta-blockers, diuretics)?

Find out whether the patient may have access to glucose lowering therapies. Be aware of factitious hypoglycaemia.

Medical History
- Have you been diagnosed with diabetes (Type 1, Type 2, or gestational diabetes)? If they are known to have diabetes, do they regularly monitor their glucose levels or have a management plan.

- Do you have any other metabolic or endocrine disorders (e.g. hyperthyroidism, Cushing's syndrome, adrenal insufficiency)?
- Do you have a history of obesity, pancreatitis, or polycystic ovary syndrome (PCOS)?
- Have you experienced any recent infections or illnesses that could affect your glucose levels?
- Do you suffer from anxiety, depression, or other mental health conditions that might affect your eating habits or glucose levels?

Family History
- Is there a family history of diabetes (Type 1, Type 2, or gestational)?
- Does anyone in your family have a history of metabolic or endocrine disorders?
- Are there any genetic conditions in your family related to glucose metabolism?

Common Causes of Glucose Disturbances [32]

Endocrine	Diabetes mellitus, gestational diabetes
	Cushing's syndrome, Acromegaly, Hyperthyroidism
	Adreno-cortical insufficiency
	Hypopituitarism

(continued)

GI	Pancreatitis, insulinoma (rare)
	Post bariatric surgery
	Dumping syndrome / post-prandial hypoglycaemia
Metabolic	Chronic kidney disease can interfere with glucose handling
	Hepatic failure can lead to a reduction in gluconeogenesis
Medication	Glucose lowering therapies e.g. insulin and sulphonylureas
	Steroids
	Beta blockers (can mask symptoms of hypoglycaemia)
	Thiazide diuretics
	Fluroquinolone antibiotics
	Anti-psychotics agents e.g. Olanzapine, Clozapine
Psychiatric	Factitious hypoglycaemia, eating disorders, stress, anxiety

Approach to Management

These questions are designed to help identify the underlying causes of abnormal glucose levels, assess risk factors, and guide appropriate testing or treatment. Depending on the answers, further diagnostic tests may be warranted [33].

Blood tests	FBC, U&E's, LFT's, TFT's, Amylase
	Fasting plasma glucose, HbA1c, Ketones
	Pituitary profile
	Arterial blood gas (if indicated)
	Auto-antibody profile (if type 1 diabetes suspected)
Other	Collecting a 'golden sample' of key blood tests is vital during an episode of hypoglycaemia where possible (glucose, cortisol, insulin, pre-insulin, ketones, IGF-1 etc.)
	Supervised 72 h fast (if insulinoma suspected)
	Prolonged OGTT (if post-prandial hypoglycaemia suspected)
Imaging	Pituitary MRI (if indicated)
	Pancreatic CT (if indicated)
	Renal ultrasound (if indicated)
Treatment	Normalise the glucose levels
	Abolish ketonaemia if present
	Treat the underlying cause
Red flags	Unexplained hypoglycaemia
	Acidosis, ketonaemia

INTERESTING FACT: The study of endocrinology can be traced back to China over 2000 years ago. Chinese healers used urine to extract pituitary and sex hormones to make medicinal remedies. The term 'diabetes' is derived from the Greek for 'siphon'—indicating the increased urinary flow ('the flesh melting into the urine') and 'mellitus', meaning sweet, like honey—which of you course will find when you taste your patient's urine [34].

References

1. Gomez-Hernandez K, Ezzat S. Clinical presentations of endocrine diseases. In: Mete O, Asa SL, editors. Endocrine pathology. Cambridge University Press; 2000. p. 1–55.
2. Junyun W, Xiling L, Xin H, Yuyan S, Peng-Fei S. Global, regional and national burden of endocrine, metabolic, blood and immune disorders 1990-2019: a systematic analysis of the Global Burden of Disease study 2019. Front Endocrinol. 2023;14. ISSN=1664-2392
3. Silverman V. Chapter 134: an overview of the endocrine system. In: Walker HK, Hall WD, Hurst JW, editors. Clinical methods: the history, physical, and laboratory examinations. 3rd ed. Boston: Butterworths; 1990.
4. Crafa A, Condorelli RA, Cannarella R, Aversa A, Calogero AE, La Vignera S. Physical examination for endocrine diseases: does it still play a role? J Clin Med. 2022;11(9):2598.
5. Can AS, Rehman A. Goiter. [Updated 2023 Aug 14]. In: StatPearls [Internet]. Treasure Island (FL): StatPearls Publishing.
6. Haugen B, Hennessey J, Wartofsky L. Goiter. J Clin Endocrinol Metab. 2013;98(1):27A–8A.
7. Latimer KM, Gunther A, Kopec M. Fatigue in adults: evaluation and management. Am Fam Physician. 2023;108(1):58–69.
8. National Institute for Health and Care Excellence. Clinical knowledge summary. Tiredness/fatigue in adults. 2021. https://cks.nice.org.uk/topics/tiredness-fatigue-in-adults/. Accessed 10 June 2024.
9. Cornuz J, Guessous I, Favrat B. Fatigue: a practical approach to diagnosis in primary care. Can Med Assoc J. 2006;174(6):765–7.
10. Huang W, Molitch ME. Evaluation and management of galactorrhea. Am Fam Physician. 2012;85(11):1073–80.
11. Darby-Stewart A. Galactorrhea. In: Encyclopedia of women's health. Boston: Springer; 2004.
12. Swerdloff RS, Ng JCM. Gynecomastia: etiology, diagnosis, and treatment x. In: Feingold KR, Anawalt B, Blackman MR, et al., editors. Endotext [Internet]. South Dartmouth; 2023.
13. BMJ Best Practice. Gynaecomastia. 2024. https://bestpractice.bmj.com/topics/en-gb/869. Accessed 3 Dec 2024.
14. Saei Ghare Naz M, Rostami Dovom M, Ramezani Tehrani F. The menstrual disturbances in endocrine disorders: a narrative review. Int J Endocrinol Metab. 2020;18(4):e106694.
15. Klein DA, Paradise SL, Reeder RM. Amenorrhea: a systematic approach to diagnosis and management. Am Fam Physician. 2019;100(1):39–48.
16. Pitts S, DiVasta AD, Gordon CM. Evaluation and management of amenorrhea. JAMA J Am Med Assoc. 2021;326(19):1962–3.
17. BAD. Hirsutism. British Association of Dermatologists; 2021. https://www.bad.org.uk/pils/hirsutism/. Accessed 4 June 2024.
18. Barrionuevo P, Nabhan M, Altayar O. Treatment options for hirsutism: a systematic review and network meta-analysis. J Clin Endocrinol Metab. 2018;103(4):1258–64.
19. Lui K, Motan T, Claman P. No. 350-Hirsutism: evaluation and treatment. J Obstet Gynaecol Can. 2017;39(11):1054–68.
20. Gessl A, Lemmens-Gruber R, Kautzky-Willer A. Thyroid disorders. Handb Exp Pharmacol. 2012;214:361–86.
21. Mingyuan S, Wei S, Qi L, Zhongqing W, Hao Z. Global scientific trends on thyroid disease in early 21st century: a bibliometric and visualized analysis. Front Endocrinol. 2024;14. ISSN=1664-2392
22. National Institute for Health and Care Excellence. Clinical Knowledge summary. Hyperthyroidism: scenario: management. 2021. https://cks.nice.org.uk/topics/hyperthyroidism/management/management/. Accessed 14 Aug 2024.
23. Garber J, Cobin R, Gharib H, et al. Clinical practice guidelines for hypothyroidism in adults: cosponsored by the American Association of Clinical Endocrinologists and the American Thyroid Association. Endocr Pract. 2012;18(6):988–1028.

24. Grant P. Erectile dysfunction: causes, risk factors & management. Nova Science Publishers; 2007. ISBN:9781619423206

25. Rajendran R, Cummings M. Erectile dysfunction: assessment and management in primary care. Prescriber. 2014;25(12):25–30.

26. McMahon CG. Current diagnosis and management of erectile dysfunction. Med J Aust. 2019;210(10):469–76.

27. Hutter AM Jr. Role of the cardiologist: clinical aspects of managing erectile dysfunction. Clin Cardiol. 2004;27(4 Suppl 1):I3–7.

28. Nigro N, Grossmann M, Chiang C, Inder WJ. Polyuria-polydipsia syndrome: a diagnostic challenge. Intern Med J. 2018;48(3):244–53. https://doi.org/10.1111/imj.13627.

29. Mahon M, Amaechi G, Slattery F. Fifteen-minute consultation: polydipsia, polyuria or both. Arch Dis Child Educ Pract. 2019;104:141–5.

30. Gubbi S, Hannah-Shmouni F, Koch CA, et al. Diagnostic testing for diabetes insipidus. In: Feingold KR, Anawalt B, Blackman MR, et al., editors. Endotext [Internet]. South Dartmouth (MA): MDText.com; 2022. https://www.ncbi.nlm.nih.gov/books/NBK537591/

31. Milne N, Di Rosa F. The diabetes review: a guide to the basics. J Diabetes Nurs. 2020;24(6)

32. Golding J, Hope SV, Chakera AJ, Puttanna A. The evolving continuum of dysglycaemia: non-diabetic hyperglycaemia in older adults. Diabet Med. 2023;40(10):e15177.

33. Pasquel FJ, Lansang MC, Dhatariya K, Umpierrez GE. Management of diabetes and hyperglycaemia in the hospital. Lancet Diabetes Endocrinol. 2021;9(3):174–88.

34. Tattersall RB. Diabetes: the biography. Oxford: Oxford University Press; 2009.

Chapter 6
Dermatology

Abstract Dermatologists will quickly inform you that the skin is the body's largest organ. As well as keeping the internal organs inside and making us look good, the skin is the site of many manifestations of underlying systemic diseases. It is crucial therefore to be able to connect skin and hair changes to constitutional upset and be able to accurately characterise and describe various dermatological disorders from rashes to lesions with clear, precise language. Additionally, an understanding of the symptoms and signs associated with skin disorders is important, as is an appreciation of potential environmental and occupational precipitants.

Keywords Rash · Dermatitis · Skin cancer · Photosensitivity · Alopecia · Urticaria · Erythema · Blisters · Ulcers · Hyperhidrosis

Introduction

Dermatology is the speciality concerning skin, hair and nail conditions, but it is important to remember how many underlying systemic diseases have external manifestations. Therefore, the medical history is critical in terms of understanding how to position the signs that are visible or existing within the skin and the larger picture and pattern of disease.

For example, signs of diabetes and heart disease can show up on the skin. Skin disorders are the fourth most frequent cause of all human disease, affecting between 30% and 70% of people worldwide. Table 6.1 summarise the common presenting complaints that you will see in day-to-day practice whilst Table 6.2 outlines the several dermatological disorders and how they can present.

P. Grant, *The Concise Guide to Medical History Taking*, https://doi.org/10.1007/978-3-031-91474-4_6

Table 6.1 Summary of common Dermatology presenting complaints and diagnoses [1]

Dermatological presenting complaints	Commonly associated conditions
Rash	Eczema (atopic dermatitis), psoriasis, contact dermatitis, drug eruptions, erythema multiforme, cellulitis.
Pruritus	Urticaria, scabies, lichen planus, liver disease, kidney disease.
Blisters	Herpes simplex, herpes zoster, pemphigus, pemphigoid
Pigmentation changes	Vitiligo, melasma, post-inflammatory hyperpigmentation, Acanthosis Nigricans, Addison's disease.
Alopecia	Alopecia areata, telogen effluvium, androgenic alopecia, tinea capitis.
Nail changes	Psoriasis, onychomycosis, clubbing, lichen planus, stress
Photosensitivity	SLE, porphyria, drug-induced, polymorphous light eruptions.
Hyperhidrosis	Primary hyperhidrosis, hyperthyroidism, phaeochromocytoma (rare), menopause.

Table 6.2 Summary table of common Dermatological conditions and associated symptoms [2]

Common dermatology conditions	Common symptoms
Eczema	Red, itchy, dry patches, often on flexural surfaces (elbows, knees).
Psoriasis	Scaly, red/silvery plaques, typically on the scalp, elbows, knees, and lower back (extensor surfaces). Pitting, discolouration, and thickening of the nails, sometimes with onycholysis (separation of the nail from the nail bed). Pustular Psoriasis = widespread pustules on erythematous skin, sometimes localised to palms and soles.
Urticaria	Hives, raised, red, itchy welts that come and go.
Drug eruptions	Widespread red or purple rashes.
Cellulitis	Diffuse, warm, red, swollen skin, usually from bacterial infection.
Rosacea	Redness, flushing and sometimes pustules, mainly on the face.
Acne vulgaris	Comedones (blackheads, whiteheads), papules, pustules, and cysts on the face, chest, and back.
Systemic lupus erythematosus (SLE)	Photosensitive rash, often on the face, across the cheeks and nose (malar/butterfly rash), scalp, and hands. Patchy hair loss, often associated with scarring.
Vitiligo	Depigmented, white patches of skin often symmetrically distributed. Potentially features of other autoimmune disorders.
Alopecia	Patchy, non-scarring hair loss on the scalp or other areas of the body.
Basal cell carcinoma	Pearly, nodular growth with rolled borders and telangiectasias (small blood vessels), often on sun-exposed skin.
Squamous cell carcinoma	Firm, scaly nodules or plaques, often on sun-damaged skin.
Melanoma	Irregular, pigmented mole or lesion that may be asymmetrical and have irregular borders.

Background History for the Dermatology System

Multiple medical conditions can affect the skin as well as medications, dietary, environmental, psychological factors can play a part, so before you get started it's useful to establish the following [3].

- History of previous skin complaints, sensitivities and allergies?
- Do you have a family history of any skin conditions, (especially Psoriasis, eczema and skin cancers) genetic or autoimmune disorders?
- Have you experienced any recent infections or illnesses?
- Do you have any chronic medical conditions? (e.g. diabetes, thyroid disorders, autoimmune diseases, liver or kidney disease)
- Medications—multiple medications affect the skin. Make sure that you get a full list of what they are taking.
- Occupation—does your job involve exposure to irritants or allergens (e.g. chemicals, solvents, metals, plants)?
- Hobbies—do you engage in activities that might expose you to allergens, irritants, or trauma (e.g. gardening, swimming, gym workouts)?
- Do you have pets, and if so, do they come into contact with your skin?
- Travel—have you recently traveled to places where you may have been exposed to new allergens, infections, or environmental factors?
- Cosmetics and skin care products—have you recently changed your soap, shampoo, detergent, or skin care products? Any known allergies to substances like latex, nickel, or preservatives in skin creams?
- Clothing—do you wear tight, synthetic, or irritant fabrics?
- How is this skin condition affecting your daily life, mental health and relationships (e.g. work, social interactions, sleep)?

By gathering detailed background information in these areas, clinicians can form a comprehensive understanding of the patient's skin condition and tailor their approach to diagnosis and treatment accordingly.

RASH = unusual changes in skin colour, feeling or texture [4]

Onset + Duration
- When did the rash first appear?
- Was the onset sudden or gradual?
- Has the rash changed over time (e.g. spreading, evolving in appearance)?
- Is the rash persistent, or does it come and go?
- Did the rash occur after any specific event, such as illness, stress, or injury?

The time course and evolution of the rash provides useful information, especially if it is tied to likely precipitants.

Location and Spread
- Where on your body did the rash first start?
- Has it spread to other areas? If so, how quickly?
- Is it localised or generalised?
- Is the rash symmetrical?

It is useful to describe the location of the rash, does it cover large areas of the body or a specific distribution such as extensor surfaces and whether it affects both sides of the body.

Characterisation
- How would you describe the appearance of the rash?
- Has the rash changed in colour or texture?
- Are there any associated lesions, such as blisters, crusts, or scabs?
- Are there any changes in the surrounding skin?

Is the rash red, raised, blistered, scaly, dry etc. and is it associated with swelling and erythema?

Associated Symptoms
- Is the rash itchy, painful, or burning?
- Do you experience any swelling, numbness, or other sensations in the affected area?

Other features of skin irritation are useful to note including which came first. Find out if there are there any systemic symptoms such as fever, chills, fatigue, or joint pain and consider could this be part of a syndrome of a systemic illness.

Aggravating and Relieving Factors
- What seems to make the rash worse?
- Have you noticed the rash worsening in certain environments or during certain times of the day?
- Did it appear after exposure to something new (e.g. cosmetics, detergents, medications, plants, or pets)? For instance, heat, cold, air conditions, friction, sunlight, specific activities.
- Does anything help relieve the rash? For example cold compresses, moisturising, specific creams, rest, anti-inflammatories etc.

Common Causes of Rashes [5]

Bacterial Infections	**Cellulitis**: a deeper bacterial infection of the skin and subcutaneous tissue, usually presenting as a red, swollen, and tender area.
	Impetigo: a contagious bacterial skin infection, often caused by *Staphylococcus aureus* or *Streptococcus pyogenes*, presenting as honey-coloured crusts.
	Scarlet Fever: a streptococcal infection associated with a fine, sandpaper-like rash, often following a sore throat.
Viral infections	**Chickenpox (Varicella)**: A highly contagious virus causing a blistering rash, usually starting on the trunk and spreading outward.
	Shingles (Herpes Zoster): reactivation of the varicella virus, causing a painful, localised rash along a dermatome.
	Measles: viral illness that starts with cold-like symptoms, followed by a widespread, red, flat rash.
	Hand, Foot, and Mouth Disease: caused by the *Coxsackievirus*, characterised by a rash on the hands, feet, and mouth sores.
Fungal Infections	**Tinea (Ringworm)**: A fungal infection presenting as a circular, red, scaly rash with clear borders.
	Candidiasis: A yeast infection (often caused by *Candida albicans*) in warm, moist areas such as skin folds, often producing a red, itchy rash.
Parasitic Infections	**Scabies**: Caused by mites burrowing into the skin, leading to intense itching and a pimple-like rash.
	Lice (Pediculosis): Infestation of the skin or scalp with lice, causing an itchy rash.
Autoimmunity	Psoriasis, SLE, Dermatomyositis.
Hypersensitivity	Atopic dermatitis, contact dermatitis, urticaria.
Endocrine	Diabetes dermopathy, acanthosis nigricans, thyroid disorders (pretibial myxoedema).
Vascular	Vasculitides, thrombocytopenia, DIC.
GI	Dermatitis herpetiformis (coeliac disease).
Psychological	Factitious Dermatitis (self-inflicted skin lesions e.g. scratching, picking).
Environmental	Sunburn, photodermatitis, heat rash, cold urticaria.
Medications	Drug eruptions, Stevens-Johnson syndrome / Toxic Epidermal Necrolysis (rare).
Paraneoplastic	Acanthosis nigricans (GI cancers), dermatomyositis (heliotrope rash), erythema gyratum repens (lung cancer), Necrolytic Migratory Erythema (glucagonoma), radiation dermatitis, chemotherapy related rashes.

Approach to Management

Along with gathering a detailed history, clinicians can form a more complete understanding of the patient's rash and potential underlying causes, guiding appropriate diagnostic tests and treatment options [6]. A thorough examination and documentation of where the rash is distributed is useful, as well as photography (consent, confidentiality and storage permitting).

Blood tests	FBC, U&E's, LFT's, TFT's
	Inflammatory markers
	Viral serologies
	Skin swabs / cultures
Imaging	Clinical photography
	CXR (if indicated)
	USS / CT abdomen (if indicated)
Other	Patch testing
	Skin biopsy
	Direct immunofluorescence
Treatment	Avoid / remove precipitants
	Topical moisturisers
	Anti-histamines
	Cool compresses
	Regular good skin care (clean and dry)
	Treat the underlying causes—topical / systemic therapies
Red flags	Paraneoplastic skin rashes
	Extensive erythematous skin rashes and haemodynamic compromise
	Necrolytic skin rashes
	Anaphylaxis with urticaria

PRURITUS = itching, the irritant sensation that makes you want to scratch [7]

Onset + Duration
- When did the itching start?
- Was it sudden or gradual?
- Is the itching constant or intermittent?
- Does it follow any specific pattern?

Can the patient identify the time course of the development of the pruritus. Does it just occur at specific time, worse at night, after bathing, at work etc.

Location and Spread
- Is the itching localised to specific areas or is it generalised?

Localised itching is more likely to be due to a focussed precipitant. All over the body suggests a systemic factor.

Severity
- On a scale of 1–10, how severe is the itching?
- Does it interfere with daily activities or sleep?

Quantifying the severity of the itch and its impact are useful guides and can help assess response to therapy.

Aggravating and Relieving Factors
- Have you noticed any factors that make the itching worse, such as heat, certain fabrics, food, stress, or medications?
- Are there any obvious triggers, environmental or situational factors.
- What helps alleviate the itching?
- Do any of the following relieve the pruritus, e.g. cold compresses, antihistamines, moisturising, specific creams).

Associated Symptoms
- Is there a rash, bumps, redness, or scaling associated with the itching? If yes, what do the skin changes look like?

Also useful to clarify if any associated rash and skin damage came before or after the pruritus. Did scratching make it worse?

- Do you experience dryness of the skin, cracking, or flaking?

- Have you noticed weight loss, night sweats, jaundice, fatigue, fever, joint pain, or swelling?

Exploring whether there is any associated underlying systemic disease is important.

Medications
- What medications are you currently taking, including over-the-counter drugs, vitamins, or supplements? Certain medications can cause itching.

- Are you using any topical products like lotions, creams, soaps, or detergents that could cause a reaction?
- Have you ever experienced itching or a rash in response to medications in the past?

Many medications can cause pruritus e.g. opioids, ACE inhibitors, diuretics.

Common Causes of Pruritus [8]

Dermatologic	Atopic dermatitis, psoriasis, scabies, contact dermatitis, urticaria.
Systemic	Liver disease (e.g. cholestasis, cirrhosis), chronic kidney disease, iron-deficiency anaemia, hyperthyroidism, diabetes, malignancies (e.g. lymphoma, leukaemia), polycythaemia rubra vera.
Drug-Related	Opioids, NSAIDs, antihypertensives.
Neurological	Multiple sclerosis, post-herpetic neuralgia.
Psychogenic	Stress, anxiety, depression.

Approach to Management

Pruritus can result from dermatologic conditions, systemic diseases, medications, or psychological factors. By gathering detailed information on these aspects, you can narrow down the differential diagnosis for pruritus and guide further investigations or management [9].

Blood tests	FBC, U&E's, LFT's, TFT's
	Iron studies
	Inflammatory markers
	Fasting glucose, HbA1c
	Hepatitis serology
Other	Skin biopsy
	Patch testing
	Skin scraping / culture
Imaging	Directed by suspicion of underlying cause
Treatment	Avoidance of triggers
	Treat the underlying cause (topical / systemic therapies)
	Anti-histamines
	Moisturising creams / emollients
	Cool compresses
	Loose fitting clothing
Red flags	Constitutional symptoms
	Immunocompromise
	Polyuria / polydipsia

BLISTERS = bubbles on the skin, small or large, filled with serous fluid [10]

Onset + Duration
- When did the blisters first appear?
- Did they develop suddenly or gradually?

Over what time period did the blisters develop and how rapidly, is useful information.

Location and Spread
- Where on the body are the blisters located?
- Are they localised or widespread?

Knowing the distribution is useful, e.g. hands, feet, mouth, mucous membranes.

Appearance
- Are the blisters filled with clear fluid, blood, or pus?
- What is the colour of the surrounding skin e.g. red, normal, discoloured?

Characterisation
- How many blisters are there, and how large are they?
- Are they small (<5 mm, vesicles) or large (>5 mm, bullae)?

Trying to quantify the number, size and type of blisters is useful for disease tracking.

- Do they rupture easily, or are they tense?
- Have the blisters spread, clustered, or appeared in a specific pattern?

Pattern of blistering is useful to recognise e.g. linear, grouped, dermatomal. Are the blisters painful, itchy, or asymptomatic?

Associated Symptoms
- Are there any accompanying skin changes, like a rash, ulcers, or scaling?
- Do the blisters leave behind scars or pigmentation once they heal?
- Is there any involvement of the mucous membranes e.g. mouth, eyes, genitals?

Do you have fever, fatigue, malaise, or other systemic symptoms?

Precipitants
- Have the blisters followed trauma, friction, or pressure?
- Was there an obvious event e.g. from new shoes or repetitive movements.
- Did the blisters appear after sun exposure or heat?

Suggesting Burns
- Any contact with chemicals, allergens, or irritants

Could chemical exposure be to blame? Have you noticed any insect bites before the blisters formed? Especially relevant if the patient has been travelling recently.

Common Causes of Blisters [11]

Dermatological	**Contact dermatitis:** exposure to allergens or irritants.
	Herpes simplex virus: causes cold sores or genital blisters.
	Varicella zoster virus: Chickenpox or shingles.
	Impetigo: Bacterial infection leading to pustules and blisters.
	Bullous pemphigoid and pemphigus: Autoimmune blistering disorders
	Epidermolysis bullosa: Genetic condition causing fragile skin and blistering
Burns	Thermal, sun exposure, friction, chemical
Metabolic	**Diabetic Bullae (Bullosis Diabeticorum):** large, painless blisters on the hands, feet, or legs, primarily seen in patients with long-standing diabetes.

Approach to Management

Blisters (vesicles and bullae) can result from a wide range of causes, involving different systems of the body. Careful questioning is required to establish the timeline and any environmental or systemic precipitants [12]. Types of blister: vesicles (<0.5 cm) vs. bullae (>0.5 cm); tense vs. flaccid.

Blood tests	FBC, U&E's, LFT's
	Autoantibody screen
	Glucose, HbA1c
Other	Skin biopsy
	Direct immunofluorescence
	Culture and sensitivity
Treatment	Protect blisters to avoid rupture and secondary infection
	Keep clean and sterile
	If blisters drained keep the protective overlying skin
	Antiseptics
	Emollients
	Topical and systemic therapy (if indicated)
	Treat the underlying cause
Red flags	Rapid progression/widespread blistering
	Involvement of lips and mouth could indicate Stevens-Johnson syndrome

PIGMENTATION CHANGES = vitiligo is an absence of pigmentation and hyperpigmentation is an excess of pigmentation [13]

Characterisation
- Where on the body did the pigmentation changes occur (e.g. face, hands, feet, mucous membranes)?
- Is the pigmentation localised (in one area) or widespread (across the body)?
- Are the changes symmetrical or asymmetrical?
- Is the pigmentation uniform in colour, or are there variations in shade?
- Is the skin texture or surface affected (e.g. rough, smooth, dry, scaly)?

Once you have established whether the skin changes are lighter or darker than the normal skin tone it is useful to note if there are any specific patterns e.g. linear, patchy, and if there is a particular distribution.

Onset + Duration
- When did it start / how long has it been going on for?
- Did the pigmentation appear suddenly or gradually over time?
- Have there been any recent changes in size, shape, or colour?

It is useful to establish whether the pigmentary changes were something that the individual was born with or have developed over time.

Associated Symptoms
- Do you experience any itching, pain, burning, or discomfort in the affected area?
- Is there any swelling, redness, or inflammation around the pigmented areas?
- Have you noticed any other skin changes, such as scaling, thickening, or blisters?

Is this part of a wider skin reaction with other features such as inflammatory changes.

Aggravating and Relieving Factors
- Have you noticed any triggers that seem to worsen or improve the pigmentation?
- Some environmental factors such as sun exposure, heat, or cold can exacerbate pigment changes.
- Have you tried any treatments or remedies? If so, did they help or make it worse?

Sun Exposure
- How much time do you spend in the sun, and what is your typical sun exposure (e.g. outdoor activities, work)?
- Have you noticed any pigmentation changes after sun exposure (e.g. tanning, dark spots)?

Clarify how long the individual spends outdoors and whether they use sunscreen regularly.

Family History
- Does anyone in your family have similar pigmentation changes or a history of skin disorders (e.g. vitiligo, melanoma)?
- Any family history of autoimmune conditions or metabolic disorders?

Helpful to clarify if there are disorders present in the family affecting the skin or systemic problems.

Common Causes of Pigmentation Changes

Dermatological	**Post-Inflammatory Hyperpigmentation (PIH):** Increased melanin production in areas of previous inflammation or injury (e.g. acne, eczema, psoriasis, burns).
	Melasma: Hyperpigmentation often seen in women, usually on the face, triggered by hormonal changes, sun exposure, or pregnancy (chloasma).
	Vitiligo: Autoimmune destruction of melanocytes leading to depigmented patches of skin.
	Pityriasis Alba: Mild hypopigmentation seen in children or adolescents, often following eczema.
	Lichen Planus: Inflammatory condition leading to hyperpigmented patches after healing.
	Tinea Versicolor: A superficial fungal infection causing hypopigmented or hyperpigmented patches, often on the trunk.
	Skin cancers: Melanoma, Lentigo maligna.
Endocrine	**Addison's Disease:** Increased melanocyte-stimulating hormone (MSH) due to adrenal insufficiency, causing diffuse or localised hyperpigmentation, especially in sun-exposed areas, creases, and mucous membranes.
	Cushing's Syndrome: Can cause hyperpigmentation in some cases, particularly in skin folds.
	Hypothyroidism: Can cause both hyperpigmentation and hypopigmentation, particularly around scars or areas of friction.
	Acanthosis Nigricans: Hyperpigmented, velvety plaques in skin folds, associated with insulin resistance.
	Diabetic Dermopathy: Brownish patches on the shins (shin spots).
GI	Haemochromatosis, dermatitis herpetiformis (Coeliac disease), Chronic liver disease
Genetic	Albinism, Cafe-au-lait spots (neurofibromatosis), Tuberous sclerosis (ash leaf spots).
Medications	Anti-malarials, Chemotherapy agents, Minocycline, Amiodarone

Approach to Management

Pigmentary changes can arise from a wide range of causes across various systems. Following the history, a detailed physical exam and appropriate investigations (e.g. skin biopsy, blood tests, Wood's lamp examination) will guide further management [14].

Blood tests	FBC, U&E's, LFT's, TFT's
	Inflammatory markers
	Fe studies
	Auto-antibody screen inc ANA and anti-TTG
	Glucose, HbA1c, OGTT
	9 AM Cortisol and Pituitary profile (if indicated)
	Genetic testing (if indicated)
Imaging	CXR (for sarcoidosis, which can cause skin and systemic pigmentation changes)
	Abdominal CT / USS scan (to check for underlying systemic diseases e.g. adrenal tumour in Addison's disease or chronic liver disease)
Treatment	Stop any offending agent
	Treat the underlying cause where possible
	Camouflage creams
Red flags	Concerns re: malignancy

ALOPECIA = hair loss or the absence of hair where it's normally found [15]

Pattern
- Where is the hair loss?
- Is the hair loss patchy, diffuse, or localised?
- Is there a distinct pattern (e.g. receding hairline, bald spots, complete baldness)?

Alopecia can occur anywhere on the body, but head hair is the most concerning to individuals. Clarify whether it is on the crown, sides, or back of the scalp and is it associated with classic male pattern hair loss (receding at the front and crown).

Onset + Duration
- When did it start / how long has it been going on for?
- Has the hair loss worsened, stabilised, or fluctuated over time?

Generally, hair loss is slow over a prolonged period of time. Sudden changes indicate a more serious or unusual cause.

Characterisation
- Are there any areas of scarring or inflammation associated with the hair loss?
- Have you noticed any changes in hair thickness, fragility, or brittleness before the hair loss started?

Getting a feel for the progression of the hair loss and any changes in hair quality is useful information.

Associated Symptoms
- Do you experience itching, pain, scaling, or redness of the scalp?
- Are there any nail changes (e.g. pitting, ridging) or other skin changes (e.g. rash, hyperpigmentation)?

These are all helpful clues as to the potential underlying causes.

Triggers
- Do you use tight hairstyles (e.g. braids, ponytails) or any hair treatments (e.g. dye, bleach, heat styling)?
- How often do you wash or style your hair?
- Do you use hair relaxers, chemical treatments, or strong shampoos?

Identify if there is a mechanical or chemical precipitant causing trauma to the hair follicles.

- Have you experienced significant physical or emotional stress (e.g. childbirth, major surgery, trauma, illness) in the past 3–6 months?

Stress is a well-recognised disruptor of hair growth.

- Have you had any significant weight changes, or are you following a restrictive diet (e.g. low-protein, vegetarian, or vegan diet)?
- Have you recently started or stopped taking any medications (e.g. chemotherapy, oral contraceptives, anticoagulants, retinoids, or beta-blockers)?

Several medications can affect hair follicle function, especially toxins such as chemotherapy which targets rapidly dividing cells.

Family History

- Is there a family history of hair loss (e.g. androgenic alopecia in parents or siblings)?
- Any family members with autoimmune or systemic conditions linked to alopecia?

Hair loss syndromes have a tendency to run in families.

Common Causes of Alopecia [16]

Dermatological	**Androgenic Alopecia (Pattern Baldness)**: is the most common cause of hair loss, caused by genetic and hormonal factors (increased sensitivity to androgens).
	Alopecia Areata: autoimmune condition where the immune system attacks hair follicles, leading to patchy hair loss.
	Tinea Capitis: fungal scalp infection, often seen in children, leading to scaly patches of hair loss.
	Traction Alopecia: hair loss caused by repeated tension or pulling on hair from tight hairstyles (e.g. braids, ponytails).
	Telogen Effluvium: stress-induced shedding due to a larger proportion of hair entering the resting (telogen) phase, often triggered by illness, surgery, or childbirth.
	Scarring Alopecia (Cicatricial Alopecia): permanent hair loss due to scarring of the hair follicles from conditions like discoid lupus erythematosus, lichen planus, or folliculitis.
Endocrine	Hypo and hyperthyroidism, PCOS, Cushing's syndrome, diabetes mellitus
Autoimmune	SLE, Scleroderma, Sarcoidosis, Vitiligo.
Nutritional	Iron, Zinc, Vitamin D, Protein deficiency.
Psychological	Stress (leading to Tellogum Effluvium), Trichotillomania (compulsive hair pulling).
Medication	Chemotherapy, radiation, anticoagulants, beta blockers, retinoids, heavy metal poisoning.

Approach to Management

Scalp examination is a good starting point to assess for any signs of scarring, inflammation, scaling or erythema. Examine the hair shafts and look for miniaturisation, brittleness, or broken hair shafts [17].

Blood tests	FBC, U&E's, LFT's, TFT's
	Iron studies
	Inflammatory markers
	Auto-antibody screen
	Vitamin D
	Androgen profile
Other	Dermatoscopy
	Scalp biopsy
	Microscopy and culture
	Hair Pull Test—gently pull on a small section of hair to assess hair fragility. If more than 10% of hairs come out, the result is positive, indicating active hair shedding.
Treatment	Avoidance of hair trauma
	Nutritional support
	Treat the underlying cause (topical or systemic therapy)
	Hair coverings e.g. wigs
	Hair transplant surgery

HYPERHIDROSIS = excess sweating / beyond normal requirements for thermoregulation [18]

Onset + Duration
- When did it start / how long has it been going on for?
- Was it sudden or gradual?
- How often do you experience excessive sweating (daily, weekly)?
- Does it happen during specific times of the day (e.g. night vs. daytime)?
- Is the sweating worse in the summer or when it's hot, or does it persist year-round?

Experience of sweating can be a subjective phenomena that can be hard to track over time.

Try to pin down the details of when a noticeable change occurred and the associated temporal, environmental, seasonal and situational factors.

Location
- Is the sweating localised or generalised?
- Does the sweating occur symmetrically on both sides of the body (e.g. both palms, both soles)?

Can the individual describe specifically where the excess sweating takes place e.g. hands, feet, armpits, face, or does it occur all over the body.

Triggers
- Are there any specific triggers?
- Do you sweat even at rest or in cool environments?
- Do you work in a hot environment or engage in strenuous physical activity that could lead to increased sweating?
- What sets off the sweating e.g. heat, stress, anxiety, physical activity, spicy foods etc.

Gustatory sweating may be a sign of diabetic autonomic neuropathy.

Impact
- How does sweating affect your daily activities?
- Does it interfere with tasks like writing, holding objects, or shaking hands?
- Any emotional or psychological impact?

Sweating can be embarrassing and interfere with work, social life, personal relationships, and impact on mood leading to anxiety and isolation.

Associated Symptoms
- Do you experience sweating at night?

Night sweats may suggest an underlying systemic condition.

- Weight loss, fever, palpitations, tremors, fatigue, or changes in bowel habit?

Assess for constitutional upset from potential underlying disorders.

Are there any signs of thyroid dysfunction (e.g. heat intolerance, weight loss, palpitations)?

Hyperthyroidism drives increases in metabolic activity.

- Do you get any symptoms of a low blood sugar such as shakiness and confusion?

Hypoglycaemia may manifest with a syndrome including sweats.

- Do you experience any symptoms such as flushing, wheeze or diarrhoea?

Consider Carcinoid syndrome.

- Have you felt extremely anxious, tremor, developed headaches or experienced palpitations?

Consider Phaeochromocytoma.

Medications
- Are you taking any medications that might cause excessive sweating as a side effect?
- Examples include anti-depressants, anti-pyretics, HRT, anti-hypertensives.
- Do you consume alcohol, nicotine, or recreational drugs?

Alcohol and drug withdrawal can cause excessive sweating.

Common Causes of Hyperhidrosis [19]

Endocrine	Hyperthyroidism
	Diabetes (hypoglycaemia, autonomic neuropathy)
	Menopause, Cushing's syndrome, Acromegaly, Phaeochromocytoma (rare).
Neurological	Autonomic dysfunction, Parkinson's disease, peripheral neuropathy
Infections	Sepsis, Tuberculosis, Malaria.
Cancer	Lymphoma, Leukaemia, Carcinoid syndrome.
Medications	Antidepressants (SSRIs, TCAs), opioids (morphine, fentanyl), antihypertensives (beta-blockers, calcium channel blockers)
	Hypoglycaemic agents (insulin, sulphonylureas)
	Hormonal medications (oestrogen, testosterone)
	Chemotherapy drugs
	Narcotic and alcohol withdrawal
Psychological	Stress, anxiety
Idiopathic	Primary Hyperhidrosis: localised excessive sweating, often affecting the palms, soles, underarms, or face, without any identifiable systemic cause.

Approach to Management

Investigations are primarily aimed at identifying underlying causes in secondary hyperhidrosis. In primary hyperhidrosis, no specific investigations may be required if history and physical exam are suggestive of the diagnosis [20].

Blood tests	FBC, U&E's, LFT's, TFT's
	Inflammatory markers
	Fasting glucose and HbA1c
	Pituitary profile
	Plasma metanephrines (if indicated)
Imaging	CXR
	CT Abdomen (if indicated)
Other	Starch-Iodine test—visualises areas of excessive sweating
	Gravimetric sweat tests—measures the amount of sweat production.
Treatment	Topical anti-perspirants
	Frequent washing and hygiene
	Avoid triggers
	Treat the underlying cause
	Anti-cholinergic medications
	Iontophoresis
	Botulinum toxin injects
	Surgical sympathectomy or sweat gland removal
Red flags	Night sweats
	Weight loss
	Features of catecholamine excess

INTERESTING FACT: Your skin makes up about 15% of your total body weight and the average adult has nearly 21 square feet of skin that contains over 11 miles of blood vessels [21].

References

1. Mian M, Silfvast-Kaiser AS, Paek SY, Kivelevitch D, Menter A. A review of the most common dermatologic conditions and their debilitating psychosocial impacts. Int Arch Intern Med. 2019;3:018.
2. Nadkarni A, et al. The most common dermatology diagnoses in the emergency department. J Am Acad Dermatol. 2016;75(6):1261–2.
3. Narayan S. Dermatological history and examination. Medicine. 2004;32(12):8–11.
4. Ely JW, Seabury Stone M. The generalized rash: part I. Differential diagnosis. Am Fam Physician. 2010;81(6):726–34.
5. Allmon A, Deane K, Martin KL. Common skin rashes in children. Am Fam Physician. 2015;92(3):211–6.

6. Ely JW, Seabury SM. The generalized rash: part II. Diagnostic approach. Am Fam Physician. 2010;81(6):735–9.
7. Tivoli YA, Rubenstein RM. Pruritus: an updated look at an old problem. J Clin Aesthet Dermatol. 2009;2(7):30–6.
8. Song J, Xian D, Yang L, Xiong X, Lai R, Zhong J. Pruritus: progress toward pathogenesis and treatment. Biomed Res Int. 2018;2018:9625936.
9. Rupert J, Honeycutt JD. Pruritus: diagnosis and management. Am Fam Physician. 2022;105(1):55–64.
10. Lakoš Jukić I, Jerković Gulin S, Marinović B. Blistering diseases in the mature patient. Clin Dermatol. 2018;36(2):231–8. https://doi.org/10.1016/j.clindermatol.2017.10.014. Epub 2017 Oct 3. PMID: 29566927.
11. Burge S, Dinny W. Blisters. In: Oxford handbook of medical dermatology. 1st ed. Oxford Medical Handbooks; 2011.
12. Michailidis L, May K, Wraight P. Blister management guidelines: collecting the evidence. Wound Pract Res. 2013;21(1).
13. Thawabteh AM, Jibreen A, Karaman D, Thawabteh A, Karaman R. Skin pigmentation types, causes and treatment-a review. Molecules. 2023;28(12):4839. https://doi.org/10.3390/molecules28124839.
14. Nautiyal A, Wairkar S. Management of hyperpigmentation: current treatments and emerging therapies. Pigment Cell Melanoma Res. 2021;34:1000–14.
15. Strazzulla LC, Wang EHC, Avila L, Lo Sicco K, Brinster N, Christiano AM, Shapiro J. Alopecia areata: disease characteristics, clinical evaluation, and new perspectives on pathogenesis. J Am Acad Dermatol. 2018;78(1):1–12.
16. Workman K, et al. Approach to the patient with hair loss. J Am Acad Dermatol. 2023;89(2):S3–8.
17. Otberg N, Shapiro J. Alopecia areata. In: Kang S, Amagai M, Bruckner AL, Enk AH, Margolis DJ, McMichael AJ, Orringer JS, editors. Fitzpatrick's dermatology. 9th ed. McGraw-Hill Education; 2019.
18. Kisielnicka A, Szczerkowska-Dobosz A, Purzycka-Bohdan D, Nowicki RJ. Hyperhidrosis: disease aetiology, classification and management in the light of modern treatment modalities. Postepy Dermatol Alergol. 2022;39(2):251–7.
19. Wohlrab J, Bechara FG, Schick C, et al. Hyperhidrosis: a central nervous dysfunction of sweat secretion. Dermatol Ther (Heidelb). 2023;13:453–63.
20. Lakraj A, Narges M, Bahman J. Hyperhidrosis: anatomy, pathophysiology and treatment with emphasis on the role of botulinum toxins. Toxins. 2013;5(4):821–40.
21. Richardson M. Understanding the structure and function of the skin. Nurs Times. 2003;99(31):46–8.

Chapter 7
Haematology

Abstract The field of haematology is relatively new, but the study of the blood has been going on for almost 400 years. The human body produces about two million red blood cells per second, and replaces 330 billion cells per day, however, disorders of the blood may be completely asymptomatic. Features of deficiency or excess of various blood constituents may only manifest at a late stage and are commonly vague and non-specific. Blood disorders themselves may be primary, due to an underlying issue with the bone marrow or component parts, or secondary, reflecting the impact of other disease processes on the haematological system (as shown for example by a disruption of Virchow's triad). Nevertheless, careful history taking is essential to clarify the time course of events, precipitants and circumstances leading to the disorder. The speed of onset of symptoms for example is central to diagnosis and may impact the speed of referral, if needed, to specialist haematology teams.

Keywords Anaemia · Neutropenia · Iron deficiency · Lymphoma · Lymphadenopathy · Bleeding · Clotting disorders · Hyperviscosity

Introduction

The study of the circulation and of its components parts relates to multiple different medical problems. Historically, clinicians used to be strong advocates of bloodletting as a way of purging disease from the body, based on the theory that the blood and other bodily humors needed to be kept in balance. However, this declined in the nineteenth century with the advent of what we like to call modern medicine.

Haematology covers a wide range of disorders including anaemia and its many underlying causes, through to enzyme deficiencies, bone marrow failure, haematological malignancies, and clotting diseases. However, there are only a relatively narrow range of presentations that the patient may report. Table 7.1 contains a summary of common presenting complaints and conditions that crop up in clinical practice most frequently are included in Table 7.2 below.

117

P. Grant, *The Concise Guide to Medical History Taking*,
https://doi.org/10.1007/978-3-031-91474-4_7

Table 7.1 Summary table of common Haematology presenting complaints and diagnoses [1]

Haematology system presenting complaints	Commonly associated conditions
Anaemia	Nutrient deficiencies e.g. Vitamin B, folate, iron. Blood loss, inherited disorders, chronic disease, medications, autoimmune disorders, malignancy, toxins.
Neutropenia	Bone marrow disorders, malignancy, autoimmune disorders, infections, medications esp. chemotherapy drugs, vitamin deficiencies.
Bleeding / Bruising	Medications e.g. Steroids, anticoagulants. Genetic disorders / clotting factor deficiencies e.g. Haemophilia. Liver disease, nutrient deficiencies e.g. Scurvy.
Lymphadenopathy	Infections, malignancy, autoimmune disorders, drug reactions.
Hyperviscosity	Blood cell disorders, such as leukaemia, polycythaemia, and thrombocytosis. Connective tissue disorders. Medications e.g. Testosterone hormone replacement.
Constitutional upset	Systemic effect of many diseases; malignancies, infections, organ failure, malnutrition.

Table 7.2 Summary table of common Haematology conditions and associated symptoms [2]

Common Haematology conditions	Common symptoms
Anaemia	Fatigue, pallor, weakness, shortness of breath, reduced exercise tolerance, light-headedness, worsening angina.
Thrombosis	Swelling, redness, and warmth in the leg, or shortness of breath.
Neutropenia	Mouth ulcers, skin infections, other recurrent infections
Bleeding disorders e.g. Haemophilia	Easy bruising, epistaxis, gum bleeding, joint pain / swelling
Lymphoma	Enlarged / painful lymph nodes, painful splenomegaly, B symptoms
Leukaemia	Fatigue, bleeding and bruising, infections, pyrexia, weight loss, lymphadenopathy.
Myeloma	Bone pain, bone fractures, anaemia, recurrent infections, hypercalcaemia, renal impairment, polycythaemia
Myelodysplasia	Pallor, dyspnoea, lethargy, recurrent infections, bruising and bleeding
Hyperviscosity	Neuropathy, epistaxis, blurred vision, headache
Constitutional upset	Fatigue, lethargy, malaise, weight loss, night sweats
Sickle cell disease	Symptoms include pain in the bones, chest, and abdomen, swollen hands and feet, and frequent infections.
Thalassaemia	Symptoms include being shorter than average and iron overload.
Haemochromatosis	Liver dysfunction, bronze skin appearance, glucose disturbances.
Polycythaemia	Bleeding, fatigue, headaches, pruritus, joint pain, splenic enlargement, dizziness, confusion, dyspnoea.

Background History for Haematology

Blood disorders can arise through multiple metabolic, haematological and environmental insults. Additionally, several medical conditions affecting the blood and clotting can run in families and a large number of dietary and medication influences can play a part, so as you explore, it's useful to check the background [3].

- History of previous medical or surgical problems affecting the blood or bone marrow and any previous investigations such as bone marrow or lymph node biopsies? Ask specifically about HIV and immunocompromise.
- Any history of GI blood loss, abnormal menstrual periods, recent trauma, pregnancies, recurrent infections, radiotherapy?
- Do they have a family history of any haematological conditions, (especially pernicious anaemia, sickle cell and thalassaemia)?
- Medications—multiple drugs, both prescribed and recreational, can impact the bone marrow and the gut (leading to GI blood loss) for example non-steroidal anti-inflammatory agents. Make sure that you get a full list of what they are taking.
- Alcohol history—this is very relevant to conditions such as macrocytic anaemia and liver disease.

ANAEMIA = reduced haemoglobin count [1]

Onset + Duration
- When did you first start experiencing symptoms of a low blood count? Were they gradual or sudden?
- Have your symptoms worsened over time, or have they stayed the same?
- Given the nature of anaemia the patient may not know the answer to these questions and the connection between the anaemia, its extent and its manifestations can be poorly related from a symptom perspective.

Fatigue and Weakness
- Do you feel more tired or weak than usual?
- How long have you been feeling this way?

Dyspnoea
- Do you experience shortness of breath, particularly with exertion? Has it worsened recently?

Dizziness or Light-Headedness
- Do you feel dizzy, lightheaded, or faint, especially when standing up quickly?

Cardiac
- Have you noticed a fast or irregular heartbeat?
- Do you experience any chest pains, especially during physical activity?

Pallor
- Have you noticed any unusual paleness in your skin or mucous membranes (e.g. inside your lips or eyelids)?

Classic features of anaemia indicate that the body is being starved of fuel to carry out its normal functions.

Diet
- Do you follow a diet low in iron-rich foods?
- How much do you eat in terms of red meat, leafy greens, fortified cereals?
- How much dairy, eggs, fish, meat, or leafy greens do you consume? Do you follow a vegan or vegetarian diet?

Consider whether they could be deficient in B12 and folate.

- Have you noticed a recent change in your appetite or eating habits?

Are they off their food through choice or is their anorexia a reflection of another underlying condition.

Gut

- Have you experienced any changes in your bowel habit?
- Both diarrhoea and constipation reflect potential bowel pathology that could lead to anaemia.
- Have you noticed any blood in your stool (black / tarry stools or visible blood)?
- Have you had any recent vomiting containing blood?

Ask about obvious revealed bleeding.

- Do you have any stomach or abdominal pain, bloating, or discomfort?

GI upset is very relevant to iron deficiency anaemia.

Menstruation

- How heavy are your periods?
- Do you experience heavy menstrual bleeding?
- How long do your periods typically last?

It's often useful to quantify what is meant by heavy periods e.g. soaking through pads / tampons, passing large clots.

- If post-menopausal, have you had any bleeding?

This is a symptom suggestive of serious underlying pathology.

Common Causes of Anaemia [4]

Haematological	Iron deficiency anaemia, haemolytic anaemia, aplastic anaemia
GI	Chronic blood loss, malabsorption syndromes e.g. Coeliac, gastric bypass surgery. Liver disease. Sub-optimal nutrition
Endocrine	Hypothyroidism, CKD leading to erythropoietin deficiency
Gynaecological	Menorrhagia, pregnancy
Autoimmune	Haemolytic anaemia, SLE, pernicious anaemia
Chronic disease	Heart failure, COPD, chronic infections e.g. Malaria, parasites
Medications	NSAIDs, anticoagulants, chemotherapy drugs

Approach to Management

Several examination features and characteristics may be present in the context of anaemia. These include pallor of the skin, nailbeds, tongue and conjunctiva, jaundice in the context of liver dysfunction and haemolysis, and clubbing and cachexia in those with an underlying malignancy. Look for koilonychia in iron deficiency and check peripheral sensation (glove and stocking) in those with B12 deficiency [5].

Blood tests	FBC, U&E's, LFT's, TFT's
	B12, folate, iron studies
	Clotting studies, group and save
	Blood film
Other	Bone marrow biopsy (if indicated)
Treatment	Hydration and nutrition
	Iron supplements
	Transfuse if compromised
	Treat the underlying cause
	Monitoring and follow up
Red flags	Splenomegaly
	Haemodynamic compromise
	Aplastic anaemia

NEUTROPENIA = abnormally low levels of white blood cells (low neutrophil count), leading to increased susceptibility to infections [6]

Onset + Duration
- When did you first notice symptoms or were you incidentally diagnosed with neutropenia?
- Was it sudden or gradual?

The patient may well be completely asymptomatic and not realise anything is untoward until the development of associated symptoms.

Infections
- Have you been feeling unwell recently, for example, fever, sore throat, flu-like symptoms, shivers?
- Have you experienced frequent or recurrent infections?
- Have you had severe infections requiring hospitalisation?

Any body system could be affected e.g. respiratory, skin, or urinary.

- Do you have unusual or severe infections? For example fungal infections.

Associated Symptoms
- Have you been getting any mouth ulcers?
- Have you had any wounds that are taking a long time to heal?

Neutropenia is related to impaired healing processes.

Medical History
- Any recent close contacts with unwell individuals?

Clarify contacts and any travel history.

- Have you undergone chemotherapy or radiation treatment recently?

Clarify the time interval and progress through the course of treatment.

- Are you taking any medications known to cause neutropenia? For example, chemotherapy drugs, antibiotics, antipsychotics, antiepileptics, NSAIDs, or immunosuppressants.
- Have you been exposed to toxic chemicals, radiation, or pesticides?

All of the above agents can cause bone marrow damage.

- Any high-risk behaviours or exposures, like unprotected sex, IV drug use, or travel to regions with endemic infections?

Constitutional Upset
- Any weight loss, night sweats, or fatigue?

Signs or symptoms suggestive of cancer or chronic severe infection.

Common Causes of Neutropenia [7]

Haematological	Bone marrow failure e.g. aplastic anaemia, myelodysplasia.
	Leukaemia – infiltration of the marrow by malignant cells
	Lymphoma – either through marrow infiltration or chemotherapy.
Infections	HIV/AIDS, CMV, EBV, Parvovirus B19
	Severe bacterial infections
Autoimmune	SLE, rheumatoid arthritis, Felty's syndrome - can cause neutrophil destruction.
Medication	Antibiotics e.g. Penicillins, sulphonamides.
	Antithyroid drugs e.g. Carbimazole
	Anti-epileptics e.g. Carbamazepine
	Immunosuppressants e.g. Methotrexate
	Chemotherapy agents e.g. Cyclophosphamide, platinum based drugs
	Chronic alcohol abuse can lead to bone marrow suppression
GI	Nutritional deficiencies e.g. B12 and folate can lead to pancytopenia
	Chronic liver disease, hypersplenism - neutrophil sequestration.

Approach to Management

The management of neutropenia will depend on the underlying cause, severity, and whether or not the patient is symptomatic or has infections [8].

- Mild neutropenia: 1000–1500/µL
- Moderate neutropenia: 500–1000/µL
- Severe neutropenia: <500/µL

Blood tests	FBC, U&E's, LFT's,
	B12, folate, iron studies, serum copper
	Blood film
	Auto-antibody screen
	HIV testing, CMV, EBV, Hepatitis serology
Other	Bone marrow biopsy (if indicated)
Imaging	CXR (if indicated)
	Chest / abdomen / pelvis USS / CT (if indicated)
Treatment	Infection prevention measures
	Neutropenic diet
	Prophylactic antibiotics
	Remove potential precipitants
	Treat infections according to local neutropenic sepsis protocols
	Ameliorate the underlying condition
	G-CSF (granulocyte Colony stimulating factor) if indicated
Red flags	Hyperpyrexia
	Severe neutropenia
	Haemodynamic compromise

BLEEDING DIATHESIS = 'a diathesis' is a constitutional predisposition or tendency toward a particular state or condition and especially one that is abnormal (in this case excess bleeding) [9]

Onset + Duration
- When did you first notice the bleeding?
- How long has it been going on for?
- Was it sudden or gradual?

It's very useful in terms of time frame and understanding the underlying cause to establish whether bleeding has occurred before or if this is the first episode.

Characteristics
- Where do you notice the bleeding?
- Have you experienced nosebleeds, gum bleeding, heavy menstrual bleeding, easy bruising, blood in the urine, or black stools?
- Is there spontaneous bleeding, or does it occur only after a specific precipitant?

Ask specifically about gums, nose, gastrointestinal tract, urine, joints, under the skin etc.

- Is the bleeding triggered by trauma, injury, or surgery?
- Is the bleeding profuse, or is it just light spotting?
- Is it continuous, or does it stop on its own?

Indicates the degree of severity of the bleeding disorder.

Associated Symptoms
- Do you get any joint pain or swelling?
Suggests haemarthrosis.

- Any history of anaemia or feeling lightheaded / fatigued due to blood loss?
- Have you ever required a blood transfusion for severe bleeding or anaemia?

Work out if the patient has been experiencing significant blood loss.

- Any recent or recurrent infections?

Recurrent infections may suggest immune disorders or bone marrow suppression.

Medications
- Are you on any medications that affect blood clotting? E.g. aspirin, warfarin, heparin, nonsteroidal anti-inflammatory drugs (NSAIDs), clopidogrel.

Family History
- Is there any history of haemophilia, von Willebrand disease, or other clotting disorders in your family?

Useful to establish if there might be a genetic component.

Common Causes of Bleeding Disorders [10]

Haematological	**Coagulation factor deficiencies** e.g. Haemophilia, von Willebrand Disease.
	Platelet disorders e.g. Immune thrombocytopenic purpura (ITP), thrombotic thrombocytopenic purpura (TTP), disseminated intravascular coagulation (DIC).
Nutritional	Vitamin K, vitamin C deficiencies
GI	Chronic liver disease due to impaired clotting factor production.
	Gastric ulcer disease
Medications	Anticoagulants and Antiplatelets
Infections	Sepsis can lead to DIC causing both clotting and bleeding
	Viral haemorrhagic diseases e.g. Dengue fever

Approach to Management

Assess potential areas of revealed bleeding, skin, joints, mucosal membranes etc. to establish the pattern and extent of bleeding. Presence of purpura suggests a platelet disorder. Patients that are haemodynamically unstable need close monitoring, resuscitation and resolution of the underlying cause [11].

Blood tests	FBC, U&E's, LFT's
	Blood film, clotting studies inc. fibrinogen levels
	Inflammatory markers
	D-dimers (if indicated)
Other	Bone marrow biopsy (if indicated)
Imaging	Upper and lower GI endoscopy (if indicated)
Treatment	Stop / avoid any precipitants
	IV access and resuscitate (if required)
	Correct the underlying cause
	Platelet transfusion (if indicated, check local guidance)
	Fresh frozen plasma (if indicated)
	Cryoprecipitate (used for haemophilia and hypofibrinogenemia)
	Blood transfusion (if indicated, check local guidance)
	Tranexamic acid to reduce bleeding (if indicated)
Red flags	Severe anaemia
	Haemodynamic instability
	Features of DIC (uncontrollable bleeding from several areas, bruising, confusion, memory loss or change of behaviour. Low platelets, raised D-dimer, prolonged PT).

LYMPHADENOPATHY = the swelling of lymph nodes [12]

Location
- Whereabouts have you felt the swollen nodes?
- Are multiple lymph nodes affected, or is it localised to one area?

Ask specifically about neck, armpits, groin, or are they generalised.

Onset + Duration
- When did it start / how long has it been going on for?

Clarify is this problem is this acute, subacute or chronic.

Characteristics
- Have the lymph nodes changed in size?
- Are they progressively enlarging?
- Are the nodes hard, rubbery, or soft?
- Fixed or mobile?
- Are the lymph nodes painful or tender to touch?

Understanding the characteristics of the lymph node enlargement helps inform potential underlying disease processes.

- Are there any overlying skin changes like redness or ulceration?

These features suggest a local infective cause.

Associated Symptoms
- Any recent or ongoing fever?
- Any issues with cough, cold, flu-like illnesses?

This could suggest infection or malignancy.

- Do you experience any night sweats?

Associated with systemic infections or malignancies like lymphoma.

- Have you been losing any weight recently?

Unintentional weight loss can indicate malignancy e.g. lymphoma, leukaemia, metastatic cancer.

- Have you been feeling tired or lethargic recently?

General marker of systemic disease.

Exposure
- Any recent travel to areas endemic for infections or close contacts?
- For example, to areas with tuberculosis or malaria?
- Exposure to animals or insect bites?

Consider cat scratch fever or Lyme disease etc.

- Any risky sexual behaviours recently?

Might suggest syphilis, HIV, or other STIs.

Common Causes of Lymphadenopathy [13]

Infections	Viral e.g. CMV, EBV, HIV, Rubella
	Bacterial e.g. Streptococcus, staphylococcal, Lyme, TB, syphilis
	Fungal e.g. Histoplasmosis, coccidioidomycosis, cryptococcosis
	Parasitic e.g. Toxoplasmosis
Malignancy	Lymphoma, Leukaemia, metastatic cancer, melanoma
Autoimmune	Rheumatoid arthritis, SLE, sarcoidosis
Medication	Phenytoin, allopurinol, antibiotics

Approach to Management

The choice of investigations and management depends on the clinical suspicion based on history and physical examination and it is essential to identify the underlying cause, whether benign, infectious, inflammatory, or malignant [14].

Blood tests	FBC, Blood film
	Inflammatory markers
	Serological testing
	Auto-antibody screening
Imaging	Ultrasound +/− FNAC or excisional biopsy
	CXR
	CT chest / abdomen / pelvis
	PET scan (if indicated)
Treatment	Treat the underlying cause
	Analgesia / anti-inflammatories if painful
Red flags	Features of sepsis
	Features of malignancy

HYPERVISCOSITY = increased thickness of the blood, causing a decrease in blood flow and leading to various systemic complications [15]

Onset + Duration
- When did it start / how long has it been going on for?
- Are the symptoms intermittent or persistent?

The patient may not experience obvious symptoms of hyperviscosity per se but may be aware of a history of previous blood problems such as polycythaemia.

Neurological
- Do you experience headaches, dizziness, or a feeling of light-headedness?
- Any history of blurred vision, double vision, hearing disturbances, or slurred speech?
- Any seizures or confusion?

These symptoms may indicate impaired blood flow to the brain (cerebral ischaemia).

Cardiovascular
- Do you experience chest pain or shortness of breath?
- Any history of palpitations, tachycardia, or fainting episodes?

Hyperviscosity can reduce oxygen delivery and impair cardiac output.

Peripheral
- Have you noticed numbness or tingling in your extremities?
  Ask about cyanosis and features of Raynaud's phenomenon.

- Do you have coldness in your hands or feet, or any signs of (bluish discolouration).
- Are you feeling more tired or weak than usual?

This may be due to reduced oxygen delivery or anaemia.

Bleeding
- Have you had any unexplained nosebleeds, gum bleeding, or easy bruising?

Hyperviscosity affects platelet function and may increase the risk of bleeding.

Precipitants
- Any history of infections, recent surgery, pregnancy or trauma that may have triggered your symptoms?

Multiple medical conditions can trigger hyperviscosity.

- Any fevers, night sweats, or weight loss?

These could indicate an underlying malignancy or chronic inflammatory condition.

- Have you been getting any bone pain or back pain?

Common in multiple myeloma and related disorders.

- Any problems with swollen lymph nodes or glands?

Suggestive of lymphoproliferative disorders.

- Any recent travel?

High altitudes—hypoxia can increase blood cell production.

Medications
- Are you taking any medications, particularly diuretics, hormone replacement therapy, immunosuppressive drugs, Erythropoietin or chemotherapy?

Cyclists and body builders may take unlicensed medications such as EPO or testosterone to improve their performance.

Common Causes of Hyperviscosity [16]

Haematological	Polycythaemia Vera, Multiple Myeloma, Leukaemia, Sickle cell disease, Thalassaemia, Spherocytosis, Waldenström's Macroglobulinemia (rare), paraproteinaemias, cryoglobulinaemias.
Cardiovascular	Dehydration, congestive cardiac failure
Respiratory	Chronic hypoxia e.g. COPD.
Rheumatological	Rheumatoid arthritis, SLE, Sjogren's syndrome.
Medications	Testosterone, erythropoietin, diuretics.

Approach to Management

The diagnosis of hyperviscosity is confirmed by measurement of elevated serum viscosity in a patient with characteristic clinical manifestations [15]. No exact diagnostic cut-off exists for serum viscosity, as different patients will have symptoms at different values. Cardiac, neurological and peripheral examination are important for identifying signs of disease.

Blood tests	FBC, U&E's, LFT's
	Blood film, clotting studies
	Inflammatory markers
	Plasma protein electrophoresis
	Arterial blood gas
Imaging	CXR
	CT head (if indicated)
	Cardiac ECHO (if indicated)
Other	Bone marrow biopsy (if indicated)
Treatment	Stop / avoid any precipitants
	Treat the underlying cause
	Consider venesection and IV hydration
	Plasmapheresis
Red flags	Neurological signs and symptoms
	Uncontrolled bleeding

INTERESTING FACT: Research has shown that mosquitoes prefer blood type O [17]. It would take 1,200,000 mosquitoes, each sucking once, to totally drain a human of blood.

References

1. Thachil J, Bates I. Approach to the diagnosis and classification of blood cell disorders. In: Dacie Lewis practical haematol, vol. 2017. Elsevier; 2017. p. 497–510.
2. Grant SJ, Jiang DC. Hematologic Disorders. In: Wasserman MR, Bakerjian D, Linnebur S, Brangman S, Cesari M, Rosen S, editors. Geriatric Medicine. Cham: Springer; 2023.
3. Milne J. History taking in patients with suspected haematological disease. BJN. 2022;31:4–212.
4. Safiri S, Kolahi AA, Noori M, et al. Burden of anemia and its underlying causes in 204 countries and territories, 1990–2019: results from the global burden of disease study 2019. J Hematol Oncol. 2021;14:185.
5. NICE. Anaemia – iron deficiency: What investigations should I arrange to confirm iron deficiency anaemia? Clinical Knowledge Summary. 2024. https://cks.nice.org.uk/topics/anaemia-iron-deficiency/diagnosis/investigations/
6. BMJ Best Practice. Assessment of neutropenia. BMJ Publishing Group; 2024. https://best-practice.bmj.com

7. NICE. Suspected sepsis: recognition, diagnosis and early management. National Institute for Health and Care excellence. 2024. https://www.nice.org.uk
8. Clarke R, Jenyon T, van Hamel Parsons V, King A. Neutropenic sepsis: management and complications. Clin Med. 2013;13(2):185–7.
9. Rubin R. Bleeding diathesis. In: Criner GJ, D'Alonzo GE, editors. Critical care study guide. New York, NY: Springer; 2002.
10. Doherty TM, Kelley A. Bleeding disorders. In: StatPearls. Treasure Island (FL): StatPearls Publishing; 2023. https://www.ncbi.nlm.nih.gov/books/NBK541050/.
11. Rossaint R, Afshari A, Bouillon B, Cerny V, Cimpoesu D, Curry N, Duranteau J, Filipescu D, Grottke O, Grønlykke L, Harrois A, Hunt BJ, Kaserer A, Komadina R, Madsen MH, Maegele M, Mora L, Riddez L, Romero CS, Samama CM, Vincent JL, Wiberg S, Spahn DR. The European guideline on management of major bleeding and coagulopathy following trauma: sixth edition. Crit Care. 2023;27(1):80.
12. Ferrer R. Lymphadenopathy: differential diagnosis and evaluation. Am Fam Physician. 1998;58(6):1313–20.
13. Gaddey HL, Riegel AM. Unexplained lymphadenopathy: evaluation and differential diagnosis. Am Fam Physician. 2016;94(11):896–903.
14. NICE. Neck lump: scenario: lymphadenopathy. Clinical Knowledge Summary. 2020. https://cks.nice.org.uk/topics/neck-lump/management/lymphadenopathy/
15. Gertz MA. Acute hyperviscosity: syndromes and management. Blood. 2018;132(13):1379–85.
16. Perez Rogers A, Estes M. Hyperviscosity syndrome. In: StatPearls [Internet]. Treasure Island (FL): StatPearls Publishing; 2023.
17. Khan SA, Kassim NFA, Webb CE, Aqueel MA, Ahmad S, Malik S, Hussain T. Human blood type influences the host-seeking behavior and fecundity of the Asian malaria vector Anopheles stephensi. Sci Rep. 2021;11(1):24298.

Chapter 8
The Renal and Urological System

Abstract The kidneys, ureters, bladder and urethra are collectively responsible for filtering the blood, reabsorbing fluid and electrolytes, forming and excreting urine. This complex waste removal system is key to maintaining homeostasis and acid-base balance so any disease or damage to its functioning can lead to serious problems, either through the accumulation of waste products and their associated toxicity (uraemia), or faults in the workings of the excretory apparatus, leading to discomfort and further damage.

Urology, also known as genitourinary surgery, is the branch of medicine that focuses on surgical and medical diseases of the urinary system and the reproductive organs. Around 40% of men over 60 years of age have lower urinary tract symptoms due to an enlarged prostate and 13% of women will experience urinary incontinence at some stage in their life. Approximately 10% of the world's adult population are affected by chronic kidney disease (CKD).

Keywords Uro-genital · Urinary tract infection (UTI) · Prostatism · Renal failure · Prostate cancer · Benign prostatic hyperplasia · Uraemia · Lower urinary tract symptoms (LUTS) · Erectile dysfunction

Introduction

The renal and urological systems are closely intertwined, and in males, the testis and prostate are important organs of relevance. The seven key functions of the urinary system are to help regulate blood pressure, to monitor and control the composition of the blood, balancing pH to maintain euphaemia, to stimulate the production of red blood cells through the release of erythropoietin, the synthesis of Vitamin D, to remove waste materials and to maintain water balance. Diseases of the renal and urological systems can disturb one or all of these functions. Table 8.1 lists the most frequently occurring presenting complaints that may come to the clinician's attention, whilst Table 8.2 summarises the symptoms that align with common renal and urological conditions.

P. Grant, *The Concise Guide to Medical History Taking*, https://doi.org/10.1007/978-3-031-91474-4_8

Table 8.1 Summary table of common presenting complaints and differential diagnoses [1]

Renal / Urological system presenting complaints	Commonly associated conditions
Renal impairment (uraemic symptoms)	Multiple medical conditions can cause renal impairment and are normally grouped into the following categories; pre-renal failure, renal failure, and post-renal failure
Lower urinary tract symptoms (LUTS)	LUTS are often caused by irritation, infection or obstruction in the urinary system e.g. UTI's, prostate enlargement, urinary obstruction, renal stones, diabetes
Dysuria	Urinary tract infections (UTI's), vaginal infections, endometriosis, urethritis, prostate enlargement, diverticulosis.
Haematuria	Renal tract stones, strenuous exercise, trauma, prostate enlargement, foreign bodies, UTI's.
Urinary frequency / polyuria	UTI's, prostate enlargement, cystitis, overactive bladder, metabolic abnormalities e.g. hypercalcaemia, diabetes, alcohol, primary polydipsia. Medications e.g. diuretics
Nocturia	UTI's, caffeine, alcohol, diabetes, reduced bladder capacity, diuretic medications, polydipsia
Urgency and urinary incontinence	Bladder or pelvic floor muscle weakness. Neurological disorders e.g. MS, Parkinson's disease, spinal injury
Urinary retention	Drugs with anti-muscarinic effects e.g. Solifenacin
Erectile dysfunction	Hypogonadism, diabetes, cardiovascular disease / atherosclerosis, hypertension, neurological disorders, psychological disorders including depression. Trauma, Peyronie's disease. Medications including antidepressants. Alcohol and narcotics e.g. Cannabis
Scrotal lump	Hydrocoele, inguinal hernia, epididymal cyst, epididymitis, varicocoele, testicular cancer

Table 8.2 Summary table of common Renal / Urological conditions and associated symptoms [2]

Common Renal / Urological conditions	Common symptoms
Renal impairment	Nausea, vomiting, fatigue, anorexia, weight loss, muscle cramps, pruritus and confusion
Urinary tract infections	Dysuria, frequency, haematuria, loin pain, pyrexia, haematuria, cloudy, strong-smelling urine, confusion, lethargy
Prostatic enlargement	Hesitancy, strangury, terminal dribbling, urinary frequency, dysuria, poor urinary flow, nocturia, urinary incontinence
Renal stones	LUTS, severe loin pain, pyrexia, haematuria, recurrent UTI's
Bladder cancer	Haematuria, LUTS, changes in urinary flow, nocturia, difficulty passing urine
Testicular cancer	Painless or painful testicular lump, change in size / shape of testicles, fluid build-up, groin pain, gynaecomastia
Bladder control problems	LUTS, urinary incontinence, nocturia, nocturnal enuresis
Hydrocoele	Painless scrotal swelling, groin discomfort, heaviness

Background History for the Renal and Urological Systems

Multiple medical conditions affect the kidneys and urological system, before you get started it's useful to establish the following [3].

- History of previous medical or surgical problems affecting the bladder, kidneys, prostate and any previous investigations such as renal tract ultrasound, cystoscopies, contrast studies, or operations such as stone removal?
- Do you have high blood pressure, heart disease, gout or diabetes?
- Volume restriction—ask about low fluid intake or gastroenteritis.
- What is your occupation? Do you have any exposure to toxins? Traditionally it used to be workers from dye factories that were at high risk of bladder cancer.
- Do they have a family history of any kidney or bladder conditions (especially kidney stones, polycystic kidneys, tubulopathies, use of dialysis)?
- Medications—multiple drugs, both prescribed e.g. NSAIDs and aminoglycosides and recreational, as well as alcohol can impact the kidneys. Make sure that you get a full list of what they are taking.

RENAL IMPAIRMENT / RENAL FAILURE = kidney function and filtering ability can deteriorate both acutely and chronically, usually measured by glomerular filtration rate and causes the development of uraemia [4]

Onset + duration
- When did it start / how long has it been going on for?
- Have you been experiencing any symptoms?

Renal failure, unless severe, is another condition that may have few manifestations despite its seriousness.

Urinary Symptoms
- Any changes in urination frequency or volume?
- Any blood in your urine or changes in urine colour?
- Any pain or burning during urination?

Find out if the patient has noticed any associated changes in urinary function.

Systemic Symptoms
- Any history of nausea, vomiting, diarrhoea or loss of appetite?

GI fluid loss can predispose to uraemia, but also renal failure can lead to GI upset and anorexia.

- Have you experienced any weight changes?

This may be linked to underlying diseases, renal cachexia, or fluid accumulation.

- Any swelling in your legs, ankles, or face?

  Reduced filtering ability can lead to fluid retention and oedema.

- Have you been experiencing fatigue?

Generic expression of underlying metabolic failure.

- Any symptoms of an infection, such as a high temperature or chills?

Explore for features of an intercurrent infection, especially in acute on chronic renal failure.

- Any recent confusion, reduced awareness, agitation, seizures?

Features of neurotoxin build up.

- Any itching?

Pruritus and skin darkening of signs of uraemic toxicity.

- Do you ever get a metallic taste in the mouth or bad breath?

Dysgeusia (bad taste in the mouth).

- Any problems with muscle cramps or weakness?

Myalgia and muscle weakness are linked to uraemic toxicity.

Medications
- Have you stopped or started any new medications recently?

Many drugs are potential nephrotoxins (including over-the-counter and herbal supplements).

Common Causes of Pre-renal Failure [5]

Cardiovascular	Ischaemic heart disease, congestive cardiac failure, impaired perfusion (shock - cardiogenic, septic, hypovolaemic).
Endocrine	Adreno-cortical insufficiency, diabetes mellitus.
Haematological	Anaemia, haemorrhage, sickle cell disease.
Vascular	Renal artery stenosis / thrombosis.

Common Causes of (Intrinsic) Renal Failure

Glomerular disease	Glomerulonephritis (various types)
Tubular injury	Acute tubular necrosis (ATN), Tubulo-interstital nephritis.
Vascular	Vasculitis e.g. Wegener's. Thrombosis. Haemolytic uraemic syndrome.

Common Causes of Post Renal (Obstructive) Failure

Urological	Renal stones, prostate enlargement, bladder tumours, urethral strictures.
Neurological	Neurogenic bladder (due to spinal cord injury or neurological diseases).
Extrinsic	Ureteral compression from external masses.

Approach to Management

There are several features of renal failure which may become apparent on examination [6]. These include ammonia smelling breath (uraemic fetor), pallor due to anaemia, cachexia, brown tinge to the skin caused by uraemic build up, and features of hypo- or hypervolaemia [7].

Blood tests	FBC, U&E's, LFT's, Bicarbonate, Calcium
	Inflammatory markers
	Urinalysis
	Arterial blood gas
Imaging	Renal tract ultrasound
	CT / MRI kidneys (if indicated)
	Renal artery doppler studies
Treatment	Stop / avoid / control precipitants
	Diet and lifestyle modifications
	Treat the underlying cause
	Regular monitoring of renal function and urine output
	Manage fluid balance and electrolytes
	Renal replacement therapy if ESRD.
Red flags	Acid-base imbalance
	Significantly low eGFR (end stage)
	Haemodynamic instability

LOWER URINARY TRACT SYMPTOMS (LUTS) = an umbrella definition that relates all the symptoms belonging to the lower urinary tract. 'Storage' symptoms are those affecting the ability to effectively store urine and 'voiding' symptoms are the ones that affect a normal stream of urine [8]

Onset + Duration
- When did it start / how long has it been going on for?
- Were there any triggering events?
- Has it been gradual or progressive?

LUTS can develop slowly over time, especially in the presence of an obstructive cause, or present very rapidly in the context of injury or infection. Clarify if any precipitants such as surgery, travel, new sexual partners etc., pre-dated the onset of symptoms.

Symptoms
- What specific symptoms are you experiencing?

Ask specifically about all of the following, frequency, urgency, nocturia, dysuria, haematuria, weak stream, incontinence.

Urinary Frequency
- How often do you urinate during the day?
- Approximately how much urine do you pass each time?
- Has the amount noticeably increased?
- Is the urine clear, light, or dark in colour?

It's helpful to quantify both the frequency and quantity of excess urination and the colour of the urine may suggest the presence of an underlying infection.

- How much water or other fluids do you drink each day?
- How many caffeinated drinks do you drink?

Does excessive intake explain the increased urinary frequency.

- Is your urinary stream weak or interrupted?

Find out how easy it is to produce a quality stream of urine and also how easy is it to stop mid-flow.

Nocturia
- How many times do you pass urine at night?

Nocturia is defined by the International Continence Society as "the complaint that the individual has to wake at night one or more times for voiding".

Dysuria
- Do you experience any **urgency**, **burning**, or **pain** when urinating?
- Have you noticed blood in your urine or other changes in urine colour or smell?

Where is the pain located and does this occur at the beginning, middle or end of urination, or throughout? What is the quality of the pain?

Prostate
- Do you have any known prostate problems (males)?
- Do you have any problems with struggling to pass urine?

Clarify any pre-existing prostate issues and treatments. This is very common in men over the age of 50.

- Do you have any problems with struggling to pass urine?

Hesitancy is the difficulty to initiate or maintain a urinary stream, whereas strangury is straining to urinate.

- Is it sometimes difficult to completely finish urinating?

Terminal dribbling is a sign of prostate enlargement.

Haematuria?
- Have you noticed any blood in your urine?
- Can you describe this?
- Is the blood bright red, dark, clots?

Timing of the presence of blood in the urine flow can indicate location.

Incontinence
- Do you experience urgency or leakage before reaching the toilet?

Urge incontinence is a sign of an irritable or unstable bladder.

- Do you ever leak urine when coughing, sneezing, exerting yourself or heavy lifting?

Stress on the bladder can lead to escape of urine.

Associated Symptoms
- Any pain in the lower abdomen or back?

Identify the location and radiation of any pains associated with urination. 'Loin to groin' pain is classic with renal colic.

- Any fever or chills?

These symptoms are common with urinary infections.

- Any changes in sexual function?

Has the individual experienced other problems such as erectile dysfunction or haematospermia?

- Any unexplained weight loss?
- Any features of anaemia?
- Have you been feeling tired or lethargic?

Look for evidence of constitutional upset.

- Have you been experiencing excessive thirst or hunger?

Consider potential causes of polydipsia.

Medical History
- Do you have a history of urinary tract infections (UTIs)?
- Have you ever had kidney stones or bladder stones?
- Do you have diabetes or other conditions that could affect bladder function?
- Do you have any neurological conditions (e.g. multiple sclerosis, Parkinson's)?
- Have you ever had pelvic surgery or radiation therapy?

Multiple pre-existing medical conditions can interfere with bladder function.

Medications
- Are you taking any medications that could affect urination?

Drugs such as diuretics, antihistamines, anticholinergics, alpha-blockers can exacerbate urinary problems, as can alcohol excess.

Common Causes of LUTS [9]

Urological	Prostate enlargement, due to benign prostatic hypertrophy (BPH) or Prostate cancer.
	Urinary tract infections, bladder outlet obstruction.
	Renal tract stones, overactive bladder.
Gynaecological	Pelvic organ collapse, post surgical scarring.
Neurological	Spinal cord injury, Parkinson's disease, multiple sclerosis, diabetes mellitus causing autonomic neuropathy.
Metabolic	Hyperosmolar symptoms of diabetes, hypercalcaemia.
Medications	Diuretics, anticholinergics, antihistamines, alpha-adrenergics.

Approach to Management

Patients need a thorough work up to facilitate assessment of the likely underlying cause for the LUTS [9, 10]. Pay attention to the abdomen and palpate for ballotable renal masses. Don't forget a rectal examination to assess the size and characteristics of the prostate gland.

Blood tests	FBC, U&E's, LFT's
	Fasting glucose, HbA1c
	Inflammatory markers
	PSA (if indicated) - before PR exam undertaken.
Urine tests	Urinalysis for signs of infection and bleeding
	Urine culture, M,C & S.
Other	**Post-Void Residual (PVR) Volume** - measure how much urine remains in the bladder after voiding. High volumes may suggest bladder outlet obstruction or neurogenic bladder.
	Urodynamic studies – tests to evaluate bladder function, including bladder capacity, contractility, and flow rate. Useful in diagnosing overactive bladder or bladder outlet obstruction
	IPSS Questionnaire - see below
Imaging	Renal tract ultrasound
	Pelvic CT scan
	Cystoscopy
	Prostate ultrasound and biopsy
Treatment	Lifestyle modification, reduce fluid, caffeine and alcohol intake
	Bladder training, timed voiding and pelvic floor exercises
	Avoid precipitants
	Treat the underlying cause.
	Specific medications e.g. alpha-blockers, 5-alpha reductase inhibitors, Beta-3 agonists, Antibiotics for UTI's (acute or chronic), diuretic adjustment.
	Catheterisation - intermittent or indwelling.
Red flags	Frank haematuria
	Anaemia
	Sepsis, acidosis

IPSS Questionnaire

The International Prostate Symptom Score (IPSS) questionnaire (Tables 8.3 and 8.4) provides a very useful quantitative measure of prostate related problems and quality of life [11]. Ask the patient to score their response to each question from 0 to 5 and then add up the total.

Ask the patient to score their response to each question from 0 to 5 as indicated and then add up the total.

Total IPSS score:	0–7 Mildly symptomatic;
	8–19 moderately symptomatic;
	20–35 severely symptomatic.

Table 8.3 IPSS Questionnaire

	Not at all	Less than 1 time in 5	Less than half the time	About half the time	More than half the time	Almost always
Incomplete emptying Over the past month, how often have you had a sensation of not emptying your bladder completely after you finish urinating?	0	1	2	3	4	5
Frequency Over the past month, how often have you had to urinate again less than two hours after you finished urinating?	0	1	2	3	4	5
Intermittency Over the past month, how often have you found you stopped and started again several times when you urinated?	0	1	2	3	4	5
Urgency Over the last month, how difficult have you found it to postpone urination?	0	1	2	3	4	5
Weak stream Over the past month, how often have you had a weak urinary stream?	0	1	2	3	4	5
Straining Over the past month, how often have you had to push or strain to begin urination?	None	1 time	2 times	3 times	4 times	5 times or more
Nocturia Over the past month, many times did you most typically get up to urinate from the time you went to bed until the time you got up in the morning?	0	1	2	3	4	5

Table 8.4 IPSS quality of life

Quality of Life due to Urinary Symptoms	Delighted	Pleased	Mostly satisfied	Mixed	Mostly dissatisfied	Unhappy	Terrible
If you were to spend the rest of your life with your urinary condition the way it is now, how would you feel about that?	0	1	2	3	4	5	6

ERECTILE DYSFUNCTION = sub-optimal erectile function in males leading often leading to problems with penetrative sex [12]

Characterisation
- Have you been having any problems getting an erection recently?
- Can you describe a bit more about what you mean by this?
- Are you still getting spontaneous erections first thing in the morning when you wake up?

What does the individual mean by erectile dysfunction. Erections tend to be less satisfactory from middle age onwards. Spontaneous morning erections are a good marker of testosterone status as levels of this hormone tend to peak first thing in the day.

Onset + Duration
- When did you first notice problems with getting or maintaining an erection?
- Was the onset sudden or gradual?
- Has the problem been continuous or does it occur intermittently?

Clarifying the time course is useful as this can tie to the underlying pathology.

Severity and Intensity
- How often do you experience difficulty with erections?
- Is the problem affecting your ability to achieve an erection, maintain it, or both?
- Can you achieve an erection during masturbation or sleep (e.g. nightime or morning erections)?
- How would you rate your ability to maintain an erection for sexual intercourse (on a scale of 1 to 10)?

It's important to establish under what conditions the ED occurs. Severity ratings provide a baseline for purposes of comparison and the impacts of any treatments.

Libido
- Has there been any change in your sexual desire (libido)?
- Do you still feel aroused, but find it difficult to achieve an erection?
- Does the issue with erections occur with different partners or in different situations?

Libido is linked to mood, situation, environmental and partner cues as well as hormonal status.

Psychological Factors
- Are there any stressors in your relationship that might affect your sexual performance?
- Are you experiencing anxiety, depression, or stress that might be affecting your sexual function?
- Have you had any recent life events (e.g. job loss, death of a loved one) that might be impacting your mental well-being?
- Have you experienced performance anxiety or fear of failure during sexual activity?
- Do you get any problems with premature ejaculation?

Getting and maintaining an erection requires significant pyschological input and there can be many interfering factors.

Hypogonadism
- Have you noticed any weight gain around your middle recently?
- Has there been any reduction in muscle mass?
- Have you noticed if you've been shaving less frequently recently?
- Have you noticed any changes in the size of your genitals recently?
- Any change in your body hair or changes in your voice?

Make sure to ask specifically about features of low testosterone that could coincide with the development of the ED.

Medical Conditions
- Do you have any chronic medical conditions such as diabetes, hypertension, heart disease, or kidney disease?
- Have you been diagnosed with any vascular conditions (e.g. atherosclerosis) or neurological disorders?
- Have you experienced any chest pain, shortness of breath, or other symptoms suggestive of heart disease?

Chronic medical conditions can affect the production and metabolism of testosterone.
Vascular conditions can affect penile blood supply.

- Have you had any pelvic or urological surgery, radiation treatment or pelvic trauma?

Consider iatrogenic damage to the penile nerve supply.

Medications
- Are you taking any medications that might affect sexual function, such as:
- **Antidepressants** (e.g. SSRIs, tricyclics)?
- **Blood pressure medications** (e.g. beta-blockers, diuretics)?
- **Hormonal treatments** (e.g. testosterone or oestrogen therapy)?
- **Anti-androgens** (e.g. medications for prostate cancer)?

- Do you use tobacco, alcohol, or recreational drugs (e.g. marijuana, cocaine)? How often?
- Have you recently started or stopped any medications that may be affecting your erections?

Many medications and narcotics can interfere with erectile function.

ED Rx

- Have you tried any treatments for erectile dysfunction before (e.g. oral medications like Viagra or Cialis, vacuum devices, injections)?
- If so, did they work, and did you experience any side effects?

Response to medications such as PDE5 inhibitors is a useful way of identifying if there is damage to the underlying erectile mechanism.

Common Causes of Erectile Dysfunction [13]

Endocrine	Hypogonadism, hypopituitarism, hyperprolactinaemia, thyroid dysfunction, diabetes
Vascular	Atherosclerosis, hypertension, peripheral vascular disease.
Urological	Peyronie's disease
Neurological	Neuropathy, Spinal cord injuries, Multiple sclerosis, Parkinson's
Medication	Anti-androgens e.g. Finasteride, Spironolactone.
	Anti-hypertensives e.g. beta blockers
	Anti-depressants e.g. SSRI's
Narcotics	Alcohol, cannabis, opioids, cocaine, tobacco.
Trauma	Surgery, physical trauma, prolonged cycle riding
Psychological	Stress, anxiety, depression, relationship issues.

Approach to Management

Getting and maintaining an erection is a complex physiological process that requires adequate blood supply, intact anatomy, high quality nervous system signalling, appropriate levels of testosterone and psychological harmony. If anything interferes with these delicate processes then ED may be the consequence. Examination is important to characterise the level of secondary sexual characteristics, size of genitals and gonads (using an orchidometer), as well undertaking a prostate and genital examination [14].

Blood tests	FBC, U&E's, LFT'S, TFT's
	9 AM Androgen profile
	Pituitary profile
	Inflammatory markers
	Lipid profile
	PSA (if indicated)
Imaging	Pituitary MRI (if indicated)
	Testicular ultrasound (if indicated)
Treatment	Treat the underlying cause where possible
	Trial of PDE5 inhibitors (if no contraindications)
	Mechanical devices e.g. vacuum pumps
	Pscyho-sexual counselling
Red flags	Testicular lumps
	Pituitary mass effects

SCROTAL LUMP = a lump, swelling or mass in the scrotum [5, 15]

Characterisation

- Can you describe the lump?
- Is it fixed in position or does it move about?
- Does it feel hard, soft, craggy?

Clarify whereabouts within the scrotum is the lump and what is its nature. Does it feel like it is full of fluid?

Onset + Duration
- When did it start / how long has it been going on for?
- Has it changed in size or shape over time?
- Any recent trauma to the area?

Figure out if this is a rapidly progressive abnormality.

Sexual History
- Are you sexually active? Any recent changes in sexual partners?
- Have you experienced any unusual discharge or lesions?

Consider whether this could be related to a sexually transmitted infection.

Associated Symptoms
- Is there any pain or discomfort associated with the lump?
- Is there evidence of inflammation, infection or constitutional upset.
- Are there any other symptoms, such as swelling, redness, or warmth?
- Any history of lymphadenopathy (swollen lymph nodes)?
- Have you experienced any fever, weight loss, or changes in appetite?
- Does the lump change with movement, exertion, coughing?

Hernias are often exacerbated by increases in intra-abdominal pressure.

Family History
- Is there a family history of testicular cancer or other scrotal conditions?
- Are there any first-degree relatives with testicular problem?

Common Causes of Scrotal Lumps [16]

Epididymal Cyst	A benign fluid-filled sac in the epididymis.
Hydrocele	Accumulation of fluid around the testicle.
Spermatocele	A cyst that contains sperm and is located near the epididymis.
Varicocele	Enlarged veins in the scrotum, often resembling a 'bag of worms'.

(continued)

Testicular tumour	Could be benign or malignant.
Infection or inflammation	Epididymitis (inflammation of the epididymis)
	Orchitis (inflammation of the testis)
Trauma	Recent injury could lead to haematoma or other issues.

Approach to Management

A scrotal lump can have various causes, ranging from benign to serious. Examination is important, including palpation of the lump to assess size, tenderness, and consistency. Check for associated signs of infection or systemic illness such as groin lymphadenopathy [17].

Blood tests	FBC, U&E's
	Inflammatory markers
	STD screen
	Viral serology for mumps (if indicated)
	Tumour markers (beta-hCG, alpha-fetoprotein, LDH)
Other	Urethral swab if any discharge
	Urinalysis for infection
Imaging	Scrotal ultrasound
Treatment	Analgesia for discomfort
	Treatment the underlying cause
	Surgical intervention if required
	Consider sperm preservation
Red flags	Hard fixed lump
	Signs of malignancy
	Features of sepsis

INTERESTING FACT: Bladder stones have plagued mankind since ancient times with the oldest stone found in an Egyptian mummy dating from circa 4800 B.C. Lithotomy has also been practiced since antiquity with accounts describing the operation as risky and difficult. Samuel Pepys the famous seventeenth century diarist, developed a bladder stone and, by the age of 25 years, realised that only surgery could deliver him from his agony. The chances of success in an age that was ignorant of sepsis were slender, but he opted for surgery. The operation, carried out through the perineum without anaesthetic by a master barber surgeon, was successful and Pepys survived. Although left sterile, he was far from impotent, and he went on to achieve fame and fortune as Secretary to the Navy and President of the Royal Society [18].

References

1. Kalantar-Zadeh K, Lockwood MB, Rhee CM, et al. Patient-centred approaches for the management of unpleasant symptoms in kidney disease. Nat Rev Nephrol. 2022;18:185–98.
2. Dirks J, Remuzzi G, Horton S, et al. Diseases of the kidney and the urinary system. In: Jamison DT, Breman JG, Measham AR, et al., editors. Disease control priorities in developing countries. 2nd ed. Washington (DC): The International Bank for Reconstruction and Development / The World Bank; 2006. Chapter 36.
3. Gottesman J, Baum N. Common urologic disorders. When to treat and when to refer. Postgrad Med. 1997;102(2):235–40, 243, 246. https://doi.org/10.3810/pgm.1997.08.297. PMID: 9270713.
4. Jacob J, Dannenhoffer J, Rutter A. Acute kidney injury. Prim Care. 2020;47(4):571–84.
5. Kellum JA, Romagnani P, Ashuntantang G, et al. Acute kidney injury. Nature Rev. 2021;7(1)
6. KDIGO. KDIGO clinical practice guideline for acute kidney injury. Kidney Int Suppl. 2012;2(1):1–138.
7. Makris K, Spanou L. Acute kidney injury: definition, pathophysiology and clinical phenotypes. Clinical Biochem Rev. 2016;37(2):85–98.
8. Abdelmoteleb H, Jefferies ER, Drake MJ. Assessment and management of male lower urinary tract symptoms (LUTS). Int J Sur. 2016;25:164–71. ISSN 1743-9191
9. NICE. LUTS in Men. 2024. https://cks.nice.org.uk/topics/luts-in-men/
10. NICE. Lower urinary tract symptoms in men: management. In: Clinical guideline [CG97]; 2015. https://www.nice.org.uk/guidance/cg97.
11. American Urological Association. IPSS Questionnaire. 1992. https://www.baus.org.uk/_userfiles/pages/files/Patients/Leaflets/IPSS.pdf
12. Grant P. Erectile dysfunction: causes, risk factors & management. Nova Science Publishers; 2007. ISBN:9781619423206.
13. Rajendran R, Cummings M. Erectile dysfunction: assessment and management in primary care. Prescriber. 2014;25(12):25–30.
14. McMahon CG. Current diagnosis and management of erectile dysfunction. Med J Aust. 2019;210(10):469–76.
15. Crawford P, Crop JA. Evaluation of scrotal masses. Am Fam Physician. 2014;89(9):723–7.
16. NICE. Scrotal pain and swelling. 2024. https://cks.nice.org.uk/topics/scrotal-pain-swelling/
17. Simons MP, van Veenendaal N, Tran HM, van den Heuvel B, et al. International guidelines for groin hernia management. Hernia. 2018;22(1):1–165.
18. Urquhart-Hay D. (1992) Samuel Pepys and his bladder stone. Br J Urol. 1992;70(5):509–13.

Chapter 9
Gynaecology and Sexual History Taking

Abstract Disorders of the female reproductive tract are common but given the delicate nature of the subject it is important to ask questions with sensitivity and respect and to be non-judgemental. Gynaecology is closely linked to sexual function, sexual activity and pregnancy, and being able to discuss these matters in a supportive and empathetic manner is crucial. In keeping with healthcare professional guidance for intimate examinations, you should always explain why any examination is necessary and what it will involve. Do this before you start, rather than as you do it. It's important to obtain consent for the examination and record this. Always offer a chaperone and note this discussion and the outcome. Make sure that you respect patient's dignity, for example, allow privacy to undress, and provide a cover for them to use.

Keywords Uro-gynaecology · Menstrual disturbance · Amenorrhoea · Sexually transmitted infections · Vaginal discharge · Fertility · Vaginal prolapse · Contraception

Introduction

The term 'gynaecology' literally means 'the science of women'. It is the speciality that supports women's reproductive health and sexual well-being. The reproductive organs produce gametes but also sex hormones that regulate the menstrual cycle as well as many other functions in the body. Table 9.1 summarises the common presenting complaints that interest the Gynaecologist. Table 9.2 lists common gynaecological conditions. 1 in 10 women of reproductive age in the UK suffer from endometriosis for example. On average it takes 8 years 10 months from the first GP visit to get a diagnosis [1].

P. Grant, *The Concise Guide to Medical History Taking*,
https://doi.org/10.1007/978-3-031-91474-4_9

Table 9.1 Summary table of common Gynaecological presenting complaints and differential diagnoses [2]

Gynaecology presenting complaints	Commonly associated conditions
Menstrual disturbances	PCOS, endometriosis, uterine polyps and fibroids, infections, perimenopause, stress, heavy exercise, eating disorders, pregnancy, hyperprolactinaemia, primary ovarian insufficiency
Vaginal discharge / bleeding	Physiological discharge, vulvitis, Infections e.g. Chlamydia, gonorrhoea, herpes, trichomonas
Pelvic pain	Pelvic inflammatory disease (PID), twisted or ruptured ovarian cyst, ectopic pregnancy, miscarriage, UTI, ruptured fallopian tube, appendicitis, constipation, IBS, psychological factors
Infertility	Premature ovarian failure, menopause, PID, thyroid disorders, PCOS, pelvic scarring post-surgery, uterine fibroids, endometriosis, medications
Prolapse	Birth trauma / large babies, obesity, age, post-menopausal loss of oestrogen, chronic pressure (coughing, straining etc)
Dyspareunia	Structural issues, pelvic organ prolapse, decreased oestrogen levels, ovarian cysts, UTI'S, STI'S, PID, bowel problems, IBS

Table 9.2 Summary table of common Gynaecological conditions and associated symptoms [3]

Common Gynaecological conditions	Common symptoms
Pregnancy	Amenorrhoea, abdominal distension, galactorrhoea, breast enlargement, mood disturbances, weight gain
Endometriosis	Pelvic and abdominal pain, abnormal bleeding, menstrual irregularities, LUTS, painful bowel movements, infertility
Polycystic ovarian syndrome (PCOS)	Irregular or absent menstruation, hirsutism, androgenic alopecia, acne, greasy skin
Sexually transmitted infections (STI)	Vaginal discharge, LUTS, inter-menstrual bleeding, genital sores, blisters or lumps, pruritus, constitutional upset
Pelvic inflammatory disorder (PID)	Lower abdominal / pelvic pain, vaginal discharge, dyspareunia, pyrexia, LUTS
Premature ovarian insufficiency	Secondary amenorrhoea, early menopause, vaginal dryness
Uterine fibroids	Heavy or irregular bleeding, infertility, and repeated pregnancy loss
Ovarian cysts	Often asymptomatic, but symptoms include pelvic pain, pain during sex, and unusually heavy periods
Ovarian cancer	Abdominal / pelvic pain and bloating, LUTS, early satiety, vaginal discharge or bleeding
Menopause	Lethargy, mood disturbances, hot flushes, sweats, amenorrhoea, vaginal dryness, low libido
Uterine prolapse	Heavy / dragging vaginal sensation, pelvic pain, symptoms of low oestrogen

Background History for Gynaecology

There are multiple medical and surgical conditions affecting the gynaecological system and it is useful to establish the following [4].

- History of previous medical or surgical problems affecting the reproductive tract and any previous investigations such as hysteroscopies or operations such as laparotomies.
- Ask about the patient's last menstrual period (LMP), gravidity (number of pregnancies), and parity (number of deliveries).
- Are they currently trying to get pregnant?
- Are you currently using contraception? It is helpful to find out what they have previously used and any particular problems with contraceptive medications or systems.
- Do they have a family history of any gynaecological conditions, (especially PCOS and gynaecological cancer).
- Have you ever had any procedures to your genitals for non-medical purposes such as cutting or burning? Female genital mutilation is illegal and needs to be documented and reported.
- Medications—multiple drugs, both prescribed and recreational, can impact the female reproductive tract and interfere with menstruation and fertility. Make sure that you get a full list of what they are taking.
- Constitutional upset—have you lost any weight recently? Have your diet or eating patterns changed?
- Ask about the patient's ideas, concerns and expectations as individuals may be very worried about fertility issues and social stigma for example.

Taking a Sexual History

For anyone that has ever attended a GUM clinic it is clear that there are some very specific and useful questions that need to be asked about sexual activities and contacts in order to clarify the potential underlying diagnosis and establish a profile of risk [5].

- Obtain permission to talk about this sensitive area, for example, May I ask you a few questions about your sexual health and sexual practices? These questions are personal, but they are important for your overall health.
- Are you currently sexually active? Are you having sex of any kind (oral, vaginal, or anal) with anyone?
- In recent months, how many sexual partners have you had? What genders have those partners been? Do your partners have sex with others as far as you know?
- Are any of your partners from overseas.
- Have you or your partners used any drugs?

- Have you paid for sex, or exchanged goods or services for sex?
- Do you used preventative measures to reduce the risks of pregnancy and infection with your partner(s)?
- Do you use these all of the time?
- When was your last sexual health screen?
- Have you ever been tested for sexually transmitted infections such as HIV?
- Have you or your current or former partners ever been diagnosed or treated for a sexually transmitted infection?
- Do you think that you might be pregnant now? When was your last period?

MENSTRUAL DISTURBANCE = an irregularity of menstruation in terms of intensity, duration, timing or complete cessation [6]

Menarche
- How old were you when you originally started having periods?
- What is the normal frequency and pattern of your periods?
- Did you go through a normal puberty as far as you know?

Clarifying at what age the individual first started menstruating is useful - as well as making sure that they did in fact experience menarche (primary vs secondary amenorrhoea) - also understand what their normal menstrual cycle is like so that you can evaluate the delta.

Cycle
- What is the normal frequency and pattern of your periods?
- How many days is your typical menstrual cycle (from the start of one period to the start of the next)?

Onset + Duration
- When was your last menstrual period (LMP)?
- When did you notice a change in your periods?
- Was this a gradual change e.g. interval gradually getting longer or shorter?
- Have you experienced any extended periods without menstruation?

The time course of change can sometimes be difficult to discern, although many women now use period tracking apps which are a useful source of data.

Characteristics
- How frequent are your periods now?
- How many days does your period last?
- How heavy is the flow (e.g. number of pads or tampons used per day, presence of clots)?
- Have you noticed any changes in the heaviness of your flow over time?

Getting periods less than every 21 days is known as **polymenorrhoea**, more than every 35 days is **oligomenorrhoea** (less than 9 periods in 12 months). Complete cessation of periods after a previously normal history of menstruation is known as secondary amenorrhoea.

- Do you have any bleeding between periods (**intermenstrual bleeding**)?
- Do you experience bleeding after intercourse (**postcoital bleeding**)?

May indicated uterine, cervical or vaginal pathology.

Associated Symptoms
- Do you experience pain during your periods?
- Is the pain mild, moderate, or severe?

- Does it interfere with your daily activities?
- When does the pain start (before, during, or after menstruation)?
- Do you experience pelvic pain at other times during the cycle (e.g. mid-cycle pain)?
- Painful periods are known as dysmenorrhea and occur on a spectrum of severity..
- Do you experience premenstrual symptoms such as bloating, breast tenderness, mood swings, or irritability?
- Have you had any hot flushes, night sweats, or vaginal dryness (suggestive of perimenopause or menopause)?

Again, gauge what is normal and what has changed for the patient. Symptoms of oestrogen withdrawal such as with the menopause or primary ovarian insufficiency can be very pronounced.

- Do you think that you could be pregnant?

Unprotected intercourse - do a pregnancy test.

Other Medical Conditions
- Do you have any known hormonal or endocrine disorders (e.g. PCOS, hypothyroidism, hyperthyroidism, diabetes)?
- Hormonal imbalances from other systems can disrupt the menstrual cycle.
- Have you had any previous gynaecological surgeries? For example fibroid removal, endometriosis treatment, hysterectomy.
- Is there a family history of menstrual irregularities, early menopause, PCOS, or gynaecological cancers

Menopausal age tends to run in families so it's worth asking if the patient knows when their mother went through the menopause.

- Do you have any chronic medical conditions?
- Are you currently taking any medications, including hormonal treatments, birth control pills, or herbal supplements?
- Have you recently started or stopped any medications (e.g. antidepressants, anticoagulants, steroids)?

Liver disease, kidney disease, chronic infections, autoimmune conditions etc. can all interfere with menstruation.

Lifestyle
- Have you experienced significant weight changes (weight gain or loss) recently?
- Do you engage in intense physical exercise or have a history of eating disorders (e.g. anorexia, bulimia)?

Hypothalamic amenorrhoea is a well-recognised phenomenon often occurring in young women who are under physical or emotional pressures.

- Are you under a lot of stress or anxiety?
- Have you been diagnosed with depression or other mental health conditions?
- Do you use alcohol, tobacco, or recreational drugs? If so, how frequently?

Common Causes of Menstrual Disorders [7]

Endocrine	Thyroid disease, hyperprolactinaemia, hypogonadism / POI, Cushing's syndrome
	Delayed puberty (if primary amenorrhoea after age 15)
Gynaecological	PCOS, endometriosis, uterine fibroids / polyps, PID
Metabolic	Chronic illness e.g. CKD, liver disease. Alcohol excess
Medication	Contraceptive medication, antidepressants, antipsychotics, anticoagulants, steroids
Psychological	Stress, anxiety, depression, eating disorders
Physiological	Pregnancy, hypothalamic amenorrhoea, intense exercise, weight loss, malnutrition
	Perimenopause / menopause

Approach to Management

A thorough medical history is essential to identify the underlying cause of menstrual disturbances. The history should focus on the pattern of menstruation, associated symptoms, medical conditions, lifestyle factors, and potential risk factors. This helps guide further diagnostic testing and management strategies [8]. BMI measurement is useful to record.

Blood tests	FBC, U&E's, LFT's, TFT's
	Anterior pituitary profile (prolactin, LH, FSH, IGF-1, 9 AM cortisol)
	Androgen profile, 17 beta Oestradiol, 17-OH progesterone, SHBG
	Beta HCG
	Inflammatory markers
	Clotting profile
Imaging	Pelvic ultrasound
	Pituitary MRI (if indicated)
	Hysteroscopy (if indicated)
Treatment	Diary (or app) to record menstrual pattern
	Analgesia for pain
	Tamoxifen if menorrhagia (if indicated)
	Treat the underlying cause
	If oestrogen deficient consider HRT (for wellbeing and bone protection)
	Consider progesterone if prolonged time with no bleeding to stimulate shedding of the endometrial lining and overcome the effects of unopposed oestrogen
Red flags	Intermenstrual bleeding
	Menorrhagia leading to anaemia
	Rapid virilisation (suggests adrenal tumour)
	Unexplained weight loss

VAGINAL DISCHARGE = discharge from the vagina - which is different to normal [9]

Characterisation
Have you noticed a change in your vaginal discharge?
Has it changed in volume?
Has it changed in colour or consistency?
Have you noticed any change in the smell of your vaginal discharge?

Vaginal discharge is normally clear and watery, depending on the woman's cycle. Changes in quantity, odour, colour (green, yellow, brown, blood-stained) and thickness of the discharge fluid can all indicate pathology.

Onset + Duration
When did it start / how long has it been going on for?
Has it been persistent or intermittent?
Does it vary with your menstrual cycle?

Useful to appreciate the time course and the relationship to the menstrual cycle.

Bleeding
Are you experiencing any abnormal vaginal bleeding?
Any recent changes in your menstrual cycle?

May indicate serious cervical or uterine pathology.

Associated Symptoms
Is the discharge associated with itching, burning, or irritation?
Have you been experiencing fevers or lethargy?
Features more suggestive of infection.
Do you have any pain during urination?
Any pain during sexual intercourse?

If dyspareunia is present consider a structural abnormality.

Precipitants
- Have you recently taken a new sexual partner?

Consider 'honeymoon cystitis'.

- Have you used any new medications or antibiotics recently?

Medications such as antibiotics can interfere with the vaginal biome.

- Any recent surgeries or procedures, especially gynaecological?

For example, IUD insertion or cervical surgery.

- Any recent use of douches, spermicides, vaginal products, new soaps, perfumes?

Can upset the vaginal environment.

- Do you tend to wear tight clothing or non-cotton underwear that might trap moisture?

Can predispose to the development of infection.

- Do you have any medical conditions such as diabetes or immune system disorders?

Common Causes of Vaginal Discharge [10]

Physiological	The nature of normal discharge may change due to factors such as ovulation, pregnancy and menopause
Infections	**Gonorrhoea and chlamydia** may present with abnormal discharge
	Bacterial vaginosis typically presents with an offensive, fishy-smelling vaginal discharge, without any associated soreness or irritation
	Trichomonas vaginalis typically presents with yellow-green, frothy discharge with associated vaginal itching and irritation
	Candidiasis (yeast infection) characterised by a thick, white, 'cottage cheese-like' discharge with intense itching and burning
Gynaecological	**Pelvic inflammatory disease (PID)** often due to untreated STIs like chlamydia or gonorrhoea, presents with abnormal discharge, fever, pelvic pain, and sometimes pain during intercourse
	Retained tampons or foreign bodies
	Cervical or endometrial cancer
Allergic	Irritation or allergy to hygiene products (e.g. soaps, douches)

Approach to Management

Vaginal discharge is a common gynaecological complaint and can have various causes, ranging from physiological to pathological. A thorough history, targeted investigations, and appropriate management are crucial for diagnosing and treating the underlying cause [11]. On external examination look for signs of irritation, redness, ulcers, or lesions. With the speculum inspect the cervix and vaginal walls for abnormalities, foreign bodies, and to assess the nature of the discharge (e.g. colour, odour, consistency) if possible.

Blood tests	FBC, U&E's, TFT's
	Inflammatory markers
Other	Vaginal swabs, M, C & S
	Biopsy for histological examination (if indicated)
Imaging	Pelvic / transvaginal ultrasound
Treatment	Hygiene advice, avoidance of douching or irritant products
	Loose, breathable, cotton underwear
	Treat the underlying cause
	Contact tracing and notification if STI
Red flags	Post menopausal bleeding
	Intermenstrual bleeding

PELVIC PAIN = pain in the lower abdomen and pelvis that can originate from the reproductive, urinary or digestive systems [12]

Characterisation
- Can you describe the pain?

Common sensations include sharp, dull, cramping, burning, pressure-like pains.

Onset + Duration
- When did the pain start / how long has it been going on for?
- Is the pain constant or does it come and go?

The timeline of the pain will help provide indications to the underlying diagnosis.

Location
- Where exactly is the pain located?
- Does it radiate?

See if they can point to the origin of the pain and any radiation e.g. lower abdomen, one side, centre, spreading to the back or legs.

Severity
- How severe is the pain?
- Has the pain changed in intensity or pattern over time?

Can the patient rate their pain from 1 to 10 and ask about what the pain limits them from doing.

Exacerbating and Relieving Factors
- Does the pain occur at specific times?

For example, during menstruation, ovulation, or intercourse.
- Does anything trigger or relieve the pain?

Ask specifically about certain positions, food, urination, defaecation, sexual activity.

Associated Symptoms
- Any changes in bowel habits, diarrhoea, constipation, bloating, nausea, vomiting, blood in your stool?

Consider gastrointestinal aetiology.

- Have you had any problems with pain during urination, increased urinary frequency, urgency, haematuria or urinary retention?

Ask about LUTS to consider a urological issue.

- Any problems with menstrual irregularities?

See section above.

- Have you had any fever, chills, or fatigue?
- Any symptoms or history of sexually transmitted infections?

Look for signs of infection or systemic illness.

Common Causes of Pelvic Pain [13]

Gynaecological	Dysmenorrhoea, Endometriosis, Ovarian Cysts, PID, Adhesions, Uterine fibroids, ectopic pregnancy, Adenomyosis
	Ovarian or endometrial malignancy
GI	Appendicitis, IBS, IBD, diverticulitis, constipation
Urological	UTI, interstitial cystitis, renal / bladder stones
Musculoskeletal	Pelvic floor dysfunction, hernias, pelvic trauma / fractures

Approach to Management

Pelvic pain can stem from multiple organ systems and the underlying causes can vary greatly so a thorough work up is required [14].

Blood tests	FBC, U&E's, Calcium
	Inflammatory markers,
	STI screening
	beta-hCG
Other	Vaginal swabs, M,C & S
	Urinalysis
	FIT test (if indicated)
Imaging	Abdominal / pelvic / transvaginal USS or CT / MRI
	Diagnostic laparoscopy (if indicated)
	Consider cystoscopy
Treatment	Analgesia
	Lifestyle modifications
	Physical therapy inc. pelvic floor exercises
	Treat the underlying causes
Red flags	Intermenstrual bleeding
	Pelvic mass
	Weight loss

INFERTILITY = the inability to become pregnant after 12 months or more of regular, unprotected sexual intercourse. It is important to consider both male and female factors [15]

Onset + Duration
- How long have you been trying to conceive for?
- Has either partner successfully been able to have children before?
- Do you time intercourse during ovulation?
- How frequently do you have intercourse?
- When did you stop using contraceptives?

Find out if the couple are actively trying to get pregnant. Have they been keeping a record, taking temperature measurements or using an app to coincide with times of likely high fertility. Are they having enough sex?

Intercourse History
- Do you time intercourse during ovulation?
- How frequently do you have intercourse?
- Any issues with sexual function?

For example ED in males and dyspareunia in females. See other sections.

- Do you use lubricants?

Some lubricants may reduce sperm motility.

- When did you stop using contraceptives?

Clarify the time frame since stopping certain contraceptives as it can be 6–12 months before things revert to normal.

Menstrual History
- As above for the female partner.

Female Details
- Do you have a history of pelvic infections or sexually transmitted infections?

Clarify when these occurred and whether they have been effectively treated.

- Any history of endometriosis, fibroids, or polycystic ovarian syndrome?
- Are you feeling pressured to get pregnant and have children?

Social and cultural pressures to get pregnant can cause significant stress.

Male History
- Any history of testicular injury, surgery or undescended testes?
- Any history of mumps or infections affecting the testes?

Testicular damage, inflammation or disease can harm sperm production.

- Do you have any features of low testosterone such as reduced muscle bulk, central weight gain, reduced shaving frequency or erectile dysfunction?
- Do you still get spontaneous morning erections?

Hypogonadism can be subtle so it is important to ask about specific features of low testosterone.

- What is your occupation?

Certain jobs such as working with toxins, pesticides, heavy metals or in a nuclear facility can impact male fertility.

Medical History
- Have you had previous fertility testing?

For example sperm analysis, ovulation tests, hormone tests.

- Have you undergone any fertility treatments previously?

IVF or Intrauterine insemination or ICSI.

- Any history of chronic conditions? Such as diabetes, thyroid disease, interfering medications?
- Have you undergone any cancer treatments?
- Any surgery, radiotherapy or chemotherapy?
- Do you consume alcohol or recreational drugs?

Alcohol and narcotics such as cannabis can cause impotence. Aske specifically are they using steroids.

- Are you over or under weight?

Extremes of BMI affect fertility.

Family History
- Any family history of genetic disorders or infertility?
- Any family members with early menopause or reproductive issues?

Medical problems affecting fertility can run in families.

Common Causes of Infertility [16]

Endocrine	Hypogonadism, hypopituitarism, hyperprolactinaemia, thyroid disorders, PCOS, premature ovarian insufficiency
Gynaecological	Anovulation, decreased ovarian reserve, ovarian failure, tubal disease, blockage, ectopic pregnancy damage
	Endometriosis, uterine fibroids, Asherman's syndrome (uterine scarring from previous interventions), cervical stenosis
Testicular disease	Mumps orchitis, trauma, cryptorchidism, varicocoele, infection, retrograde ejaculation. Heat exposure, hot baths can denature sperm
Lifestyle factors	Drugs, smoking, alcohol, obesity, excessive exercise, stress
Psychological	Mental health problems e.g. anxiety, depression

Approach to Management

Infertility is defined as the inability to conceive after 12 months of regular, unprotected intercourse (6 months if the woman is over 35 years of age). Questions, examination and investigations should focus on both male and female partners. In about 10–15% of couples, the cause of infertility is never identified [17].

Blood tests	FBC, U&E's, LFT's, TFT's
	Inflammatory markers
	Anterior pituitary profile
	Androgen profile, Oestradiol, anti-Mullerian hormone (AMH)
	Mid-luteal progesterone levels (confirm ovulation)
Other	Semen analysis
	Genetic testing (if indicated)
	Testicular biopsy
Imaging	Abdominal / pelvic ultrasound
	Hysterosalpingography
	Diagnostic laparoscopy
	Endometrial biopsy (if indicated)
	Scrotal ultrasound (in males)
Treatment	Manage the underlying cause
	Lifestyle and weight management
	Diet and exercise
	Stress reduction
	Consider ovulation induction with clomiphene / Letrozole
	Consider exogenous gonadotrophins
	Assisted reproductive technologies
Red flags	Pituitary mass effect
	Pelvic masses
	Scrotal masses

PROLAPSE = vaginal or uterine descent, commonly occurring when the pelvic floor muscles and ligaments become weak [18]

Characterisation
- Have you noticed a bulge, a pressure or a protrusion from your vagina?
- Can you see or feel anything?

Patient's often describe the sensation of 'something coming down' or 'dragging' in their vagina.

Onset + Duration
- When did it start / how long has it been going on for?
- Has the sensation worsened over time?

Has this been developing very slowly or did something suddenly change.

Severity
- Is it painful?
- Is there discomfort or pain, especially during activities such as standing or walking?
- Do your symptoms worsen at the end of the day or with prolonged standing?

Find out whether the prolapse interfere with day-to-day activities.

Triggers
- Do you have any history of heavy lifting or work that requires straining?
- Do you have a history of chronic cough, asthma, or respiratory conditions that increase abdominal pressure?

Consider anything that might place increased strain and pressure on the pelvic floor muscles and suspensory ligaments in the pelvis.

- Do you suffer from chronic constipation, or have you noticed straining during bowel movements?

Associated Symptoms
- Any changes in urinary control or bladder emptying?

Has the patient had any problems with urinary incontinence, urgency, or frequency.

- Do you have difficulty with bowel movements?

Does it cause problems with constipation, tenesmus or incomplete evacuation.

- Do you experience any difficulty with sexual intercourse?

Prolapse can interfere with penetrative sex?

- Do you experience vaginal bleeding or spotting?

Damage to the vaginal or uterine structures may precipitate bleeding.

- Do you experience back pain or discomfort?

Are there other structural weaknesses in the neighbourhood.

Obs/Gynae History
- How many children have you given birth to, and were they delivered vaginally or via caesarean section?
- Did you experience any complications during childbirth e.g. prolonged labour, use of forceps or vacuum, or a large baby?
- Have you had any pelvic surgeries?

Consider anything traumatic that could have damaged pelvic anatomy.

- Are you menopausal, and if so, at what age did menopause occur?

Low oestrogen status can affect the strength and elasticity of connective tissues, muscles and ligaments.

Common Causes of Prolapse [19]

Musculoskeletal	Childbirth trauma, pelvic surgery, pelvic floor weakness
	Exacerbated by chronic cough, obesity and exertion
GI	Chronic constipation, chronic straining
Neurological	Multiple sclerosis, spinal cord injury
Endocrine	Menopause, hypogonadism

Approach to Management

Pelvic Examination is key to diagnosing the extent of the prolapse. The patient is often examined while standing, and the degree of prolapse is assessed using the **Pelvic Organ Prolapse Quantification System (POP-Q)** [20], which grades the prolapse on a scale from;

0 = No prolapse
1 = Most distal portion of the prolapse is more than 1 cm above the level of hymen.
2 = Most distal portion of the prolapse is 1 cm or less proximal or distal to the hymen.
3 = The uterus protrudes halfway out of the vagina.
4 = Complete prolapse.

The Valsalva manoeuvre can help to reveal a prolapse that may not be apparent at rest.

Blood tests	N/A
Imaging	Pelvic / abdominal ultrasound or MRI scan
Other	Urinalysis to check for infections or other urinary abnormalities
	Urodynamic testing may be done if the patient has urinary symptoms like incontinence or urgency, to assess bladder function
	Post-void residual (PVR) volume
Treatment	Pelvic floor exercises
	Pessary devices to support the pelvic organs
	Avoid straining and heavy lifting
	Surgical repair
	Weight loss
	Consider HRT and topical oestrogen creams
Red flags	Post-menopausal bleeding
	Pelvic masses

DYSPAREUNIA = painful sexual intercourse. It affects both men and women, although it is more common in women [21]

Onset + Duration
- When did the pain during intercourse first begin?
- Has it been present since your first sexual experience, or did it develop later?
- Is it continuous, or does it come and go?

Time frame is important and clarify whether this is primary or secondary dyspareunia.

Nature and Location
- Is the pain located at the vaginal opening (superficial) or deeper inside (deep dyspareunia)?
- Can you describe the pain?
- Is the pain associated with penetration or deep thrusting?
- Do you experience pain during other activities like tampon insertion or pelvic examinations?

Assess whether this is superficial or deep dyspareunia and what the sensation is actually like burning, stabbing, aching etc.

Triggers
- Does the pain occur with every sexual encounter or only in certain situations?
- Is the pain worse in specific positions or with specific partners?
- Is the pain related to your menstrual cycle?
- Do you experience pain at other times (e.g. urination, bowel movements)?

Can the patient identify any particular precipitants or associations, is it worse before or after their period and does similar pain occur on other occasions, for example whilst going to the toilet.

Associated Symptoms
- Do you experience vaginal dryness, itching, or discharge?
- Any history of abnormal vaginal bleeding or spotting?

Are there features of vaginal pathology, infection or low oestrogen.

- Any pelvic pain, low back pain, or abdominal pain outside of sexual activity?
- Does the pain radiate or occur when not having sex?
- Any urinary symptoms?

Ask about LUTS to see if there are signs of infection.

- Any difficulties with lubrication or hormonal changes?

Could the patient be peri-menopausal?

- Do you have a history of sexually transmitted infections (STI's)?

Find out if the individual prone to sexually related diseases.

Psychological Factors
- How is your emotional relationship with your partner?
- Do you feel anxious or stressed about sex?
- Any history of sexual abuse or trauma?
- Are there any significant life stressors affecting your overall well-being?

Sex can be a deeply psychological interaction and be subject to a variety of stimulants and stressors. What is happening in the individual's life?

Medications
- Are you using any medications that could affect libido or cause vaginal dryness?

Ask about antihistamines, antidepressants, hormonal therapies.

Common Causes of Dyspareunia [21]

Gynaecological	Vulvovaginitis, vulvodynia, vaginal dryness, PID, Endometriosis, Uterine fibroids, Ovarian cysts, vaginismus
Urological	UTI's, Interstitial cystitis
GI	IBS, IBD
Neurological	Pelvic Nerve Entrapment, Pudendal neuralgia
Musculo-skeletal	Postpartum or Post-Surgical Changes, Pelvic floor dysfunction
Psychological	Anxiety, depression, stress, history of trauma or abuse

Approach to Management

The approach to dyspareunia includes a detailed medical history, careful gynaecological / pelvic examination, identifying underlying causes, working through the appropriate investigations, and treating both symptoms and the underlying aetiology [22].

Blood tests	FBC, U&U's, LFT's, TFT's
	Glucose, HbA1c
	Inflammatory markers
	STD screen
	Oestrogen, LH, FSH
Other	Vaginal swab
	M,C & S
	Urinalysis
	Urodynamic studies (if bladder involvement suspected)
Imaging	Pelvic / transvaginal ultrasound
	Pelvic MRI (if indicated)
	Diagnostic laparoscopy

(continued)

Treatment	Analgesia
	Stress reduction / relaxation techniques
	Use of lubricating agents
	Topical oestrogen creams
	Muscle relaxants
	Pelvic floor exercises
	Counselling / sex therapy / CBT
	Treat the underlying cause
Red flags	Severe vaginal muscle spasm
	Bleeding post intercourse

INTERESTING FACT: In ancient civilizations, such as Egypt, Greece, and Rome, women's health and childbirth were often managed by female practitioners known as "midwives" or "wise women" and this has continued throughout history. These women were skilled in the art of childbirth and were responsible for delivering babies, as well as providing prenatal and postnatal care to women. Independently knowledgeable healers and practitioners threatened paternalistic society and the medical hierarchy and were often burnt as witches [23]. In the modern US, midwives are often seen as both an anathema and a commercial threat to the lucrative obstetric medical-industrial complex.

References

1. De Corte P, Klinghardt M, von Stockum S, Heinemann K. Time to diagnose endometriosis: current status, challenges and regional characteristics—a systematic literature review. BJOG. 2025;132:118–30.
2. von Glehn MP, Sidon LU, Machado ER. Gynecological complaints and their associated factors among women in a family health-care clinic. J Family Med Prim Care. 2017;6(1):88–92.
3. Apoola A. Common Gynaecological problems. Sex Transm Infect. 2000;76(1):60–1.
4. Unkels, R. Gynaecological history taking and examination. 2008. https://www.glowm.com/pdf/Chap-01_Unkels.pdf
5. Centres for Disease Control. A Guide to Taking a Sexual History. 2024. https://www.cdc.gov/std/treatment/sexualhistory.pdf
6. Saei Ghare Naz M, Rostami Dovom M, Ramezani TF. The menstrual disturbances in endocrine disorders: a narrative review. Int J Endocrinol Metab. 2020;18(4):e106694.
7. Klein DA, Paradise SL, Reeder RM. Amenorrhea: a systematic approach to diagnosis and management. Am Fam Physician. 2019;100(1):39–48.
8. Pitts S, DiVasta AD, Gordon CM. Evaluation and management of amenorrhea. J American Med Assoc (JAMA). 2021;326(19):1962–3.
9. BASHH. Standards for the management of sexually transmitted infections (STIs). British Association of Sexual Health and HIV. 2019. http://www.bashh.org
10. Rao V, Mahmood T. Vaginal discharge. Obst Gynaecol Reprod Med. 2020;30(1):11–8.
11. NICE. Vaginal discharge. 2024. https://cks.nice.org.uk/topics/vaginal-discharge/
12. European Association of Urology. Chronic pelvic pain. 2024. https://uroweb.org/guidelines/chronic-pelvic-pain

13. Franco PN, García-Baizán A, Aymerich M, Maino C, Frade-Santos S, Ippolito D, Otero-García M. Gynaecological causes of acute pelvic pain: common and not-so-common imaging findings. Life (Basel). 2023;13(10):2025.
14. Kruszka PS, Kruszka SJ. Evaluation of acute pelvic pain in women. Am Fam Physician. 2010;82(2):141–7.
15. WHO. Infertility. World Health Organisation. 2023. http://www.who.int
16. Gnoth C, Godehardt E, Frank-Herrmann P, et al. Definition and prevalence of subfertility and infertility. Hum Reprod. 2005;20(5):1144–7.
17. BMJ Best Practice. Infertility in women. BMJ Publishing Group; 2023. http://bestpractice.bmj.com
18. Iglesia CB, Smithling KR. Pelvic organ prolapse. Am Fam Physician. 2017;96(3):179–85.
19. Aboseif C, Liu P. Pelvic Organ Prolapse. [Updated 2022 Oct 3]. In: StatPearls [Internet]. Treasure Island (FL): StatPearls Publishing; 2025. Available from: https://www.ncbi.nlm.nih.gov/books/NBK563229/
20. Persu C, Chapple CR, Cauni V, Gutue S, Geavlete P. Pelvic organ prolapse quantification system (POP-Q) – a new era in pelvic prolapse staging. J Med Life. 2011;4(1):75–81.
21. Heim LJ. Evaluation and differential diagnosis of dyspareunia. Am Fam Physician. 2001;63(8):1535–44.
22. Morris C, Briggs C, Navani M. Dyspareunia. InnovAiT. 2021;14(10):607–14.
23. Towler J, Bramall J. Midwives in history and society. 1st ed. Routledge; 1986.

Chapter 10
The Musculo-Skeletal System

Abstract The musculo-skeletal system covers the bones, joints and connective tissues that control and support our movement and day to day functions. As well as local injury, infection and inflammation, a wide variety of systemic diseases can affect the locomotor system and result in compromised health and wellbeing. Autoimmune conditions for example can attack the joints, causing a mono- or poly-arthropathy, but also the skin and other organ systems (known as extra-articular manifestations). Approximately 18 million people worldwide are living with rheumatoid arthritis. Because rheumatological disorders also affect blood vessels, organs and a host of other body parts, rheumatologist need to delve down into the effects on those systems as well.

Given the impact that MSK conditions can have on patients, especially pain and function, it is important to establish what problems they are facing, their limitations and what they want to achieve from medical intervention and be mindful of the psychological impacts of such disorders.

Keywords Auto-immune disease · Rheumatic disease · Orthopaedics · Arthritis · Arthropathy · Joint disease · Acute hot joint · Back pain

Introduction

Musculo-skeletal (MSK) disorders and joint problems are commonly dealt with by Rheumatologists, Orthopaedic surgeons and expert Physiotherapists. These conditions can have major impacts on functional abilities, day to day activities and overall quality of life. A great deal of research suggests that a holistic approach to managing these diseases is more effective than the traditional biomedical model alone [1]. Consideration therefore needs to be given to not only pain relief and reducing inflammation, but also on complementary care including exercise therapies,

P. Grant, *The Concise Guide to Medical History Taking*, https://doi.org/10.1007/978-3-031-91474-4_10

Table 10.1 Summary table of common MSK presenting complaints and differential diagnoses [2]

Musculo-skeletal system presenting complaints	Commonly associated conditions
Joint pain (arthralgia)	Rheumatoid arthritis, gout, osteoarthritis, fractures, psoriatic arthritis, ankylosing spondylitis
Joint swelling (effusion)	Rheumatoid arthritis, gout, reactive arthritis, septic arthritis, haemarthrosis, trauma / sprains
Joint deformity	Rheumatoid arthritis, psoriatic arthritis, osteoarthritis, congenital abnormalities, trauma / dislocations, Charcot joint
Joint stiffness	Rheumatoid arthritis, psoriatic arthritis, osteoarthritis, fractures or sprains
Back pain	Mechanical causes—strain / sprain, ankylosing spondylitis, trauma / fractures, whiplash, metastatic cancer, multiple myeloma, sciatica, spinal stenosis
Fatigue	Systemic inflammatory diseases, rheumatoid arthritis, fibromyalgia, stress, depression, hypothyroidism, SLE, Anaemia
Polyarthropathy	Rheumatoid arthritis, still's disease, HSP, psoriatic arthritis, SLE, sarcoidosis, scleroderma, Sjogren's syndrome, Lyme disease, paraneoplastic syndrome

optimising nutrition, education and self-awareness, social support, constructive coping strategies and wellness aspects such as meditation, mindfulness and sleep quality. Table 10.1 summarises common conditions and Table 10.2 lists common MSK diseases and their associated symptoms.

Background History for the Musculo-Skeletal System

A host of local and systemic conditions affect the muscle-skeletal system and a large number of dietary and environmental factors can play a part. The background history of factors influencing the MSK system are useful to understand before you get started on the specifics [4].

- History of pre-existing medical or surgical problems affecting the joints, chronic diseases, autoimmune conditions and any recent infections (including sexually transmitted).
- Any previous investigations such as joint aspirations or operations such as joint replacements?
- Do they have a family history of any autoimmune conditions (especially RA in first degree relatives) or joint conditions?

Table 10.2 Summary table of common MSK conditions and associated symptoms [3]

Common MSK conditions	Common symptoms
Rheumatoid arthritis	Pain, aching, or stiffness in the joints, especially in the morning. Reduced mobility, fatigue, weight loss.
Osteoarthritis	Joint pain, joint stiffness, especially in the morning or after resting, that usually lasts less than 30 minutes. Reduced range of movement
Septic arthritis	Severe joint pain. Swelling, redness and warmth. Pyrexia
Bursitis	Dull achy pain in the joint, worse with pressure. Joint swelling, warmth and stiffness
Fibromyalgia	Muscle pain and tenderness - mainly between the joints. Fatigue, sleep disturbance, extreme sensitivity
Joint fracture	Swelling, bruising, bleeding, pain, warmth, deformity, limited range of movement
Osteoporosis	Bone pain, loss of height, stooped posture, back pain
Scoliosis	Visibly curved spine, uneven shoulders or hips, uneven leg length
Seronegative spondyloarthropathy	Pain, stiffness, and swelling in the lower back, hips, shoulders, knees, and elbows. Prolonged morning stiffness
Gout	Joint pain, redness, swelling, warmth, tenderness, pyrexia, malaise
Polymyalgia Rheumatica	Pain and stiffness in the muscles of the shoulders, neck, hips, and upper arms
Tendonitis	Pain in a tendon that gets worse on movement, grating or crackling sensation, swelling, warmth, redness
Systemic lupus erythematosus	Arthritis, fevers, fatigue, rashes including on the face, constitutional upset, chest pain

- Medications—multiple drugs, can impact the gut. Make sure that you get a full list of what they are taking, including use of NSAIDs as these can increase the risks of upper GI bleeding.
- Do they use intravenous drugs—this is a risk factor for septic arthritis.
- Constitutional upset—have you lost any weight recently? Have your diet or eating patterns changed?
- What do you do for a living? Certain occupations and activities are associated with joint wear and tear and specific MSK conditions e.g. carpet-fitters knee, a form of bursitis.
- Social context—what is their home environment like? Do they live on one or two floors. What is your level of physical activity? Can they independently mobilise and manage with activities of daily living or do they need help?

JOINT PROBLEMS = there is a concatenation of signs and symptoms that appear with disease of the joints that includes pain, swelling, deformity, stiffness and instability [5]

Characterisation
- Can you describe what has happened to your joints?
- How many / which specific joints are affected?
- Is the pain sharp, dull, constant, or intermittent?

Establish the patient's overview of their joint problems and the distribution before going into more specifics.

Onset + Duration
- When did it start / how long has it been going on for?
- Has this been sudden or gradual?
- Does the problem come and go?
- Have things been progressively worsening over time?
- Is there any history of recent trauma?

Is this something that has been grumbling away for years suggesting a more benign cause or a very rapid development?

Joint Pain
- Is the pain inside the joint itself or around the joint?
- Can you point to where the pain is located?
- Does the pain spread anywhere else?

Find out more about the nature of the pain.

- How severe is the pain on a scale of 1–10?

Ask the patient to quantify the intensity of their pain and describe the impact this has on their quality of life.

- Does anything make the pain better or worse?

What are the exacerbating and relieving factors; rest, movement, analgesia, hot baths etc.

Joint Swelling
- Is there noticeable swelling?
- Does the joint feel warm?
- Have you noticed any associated redness of the skin overlying the swollen joints?

Warmth and swelling are features of rheumatological conditions causing inflammation within the joint space. If there is joint swelling and fever this requires urgent review.

Joint Stiffness

- Do your joints feel stiff?
- Joint stiffness is commonly associated with rheumatological joint pain.
- Do you get stiffness at any particular time of day?
- How long does morning stiffness last for?

Morning stiffness occurs with several types of joint disorder. OA is common with ageing and tends to resolve within 30 minutes of movement. RA and psoriatic arthritis can last longer than 30 minutes.

Joint Deformity

- Have any of your joints lost their shape or become disfigured?

Confirm on examination which joints are affected and the type(s) or deformity e.g. swan's neck, mallet finger, ulnar drift etc.

- Have you noticed any lumps around your joints?

For example, Bouchard's and Heberden's nodes.

- Is the joint unstable?
- Does it feel like it is coming apart?

Joint instability is a sign of wear and tear, dislocation or hypermobility.

Associated Symptoms

- Does it interfere with daily activities?

It is useful to record what the patient is no longer able to do, or wants to do, as this can be used as a therapeutic goal.

- Are you experiencing fever, sweats, weight loss, or fatigue?

Are there features of systemic or constitutional upset.

- Have you noticed any skin rashes or nail changes?

Plaques on extensor surfaces and nail changes such as onycholysis suggest psoriasis.

- Any eye irritation or redness?
- Have you experienced very dry eyes?
- Do you have any breathing or lung problems?
- Any problems / discomfort with passing urine—or any discharge?

Extra-articular manifestations of rheumatological disease include uveitis (ankylosing spondylitis), dry eyes (Sjogren's syndrome), interstitial lung disease (both RA and SLE) and urethritis (reactive arthritis).

Common Causes of Joint Disorders [6]

Musculo-skeletal	Osteoarthritis, Tendonitis, Bursitis, Trauma (fracture / dislocations)
Auto-immune	Rheumatoid arthritis, psoriatic arthritis, SLE, Sjogren's, ankylosing spondylitis, juvenile arthritis
Metabolic	Gout, Pseudogout
Infectious	Septic arthritis, Lyme disease, parvovirus, viral hepatitis
Neurological	Nerve pathology, injury, compression

Approach to Management

A clear framework is required to establish the pattern / distribution / symmetry of joint disease and its development, as well as the functional impact. Inspect, feel and move the joints to assess for their range of movement. Check for lymphadenopathy and other signs of local / systemic inflammation [4, 6].

Blood tests	FBC, U&E's, LFT's
	Uric acid levels
	Inflammatory markers
	Auto-immune profile e.g. Rheumatoid factor and anti-CCP AB's.
	ANA, ANCA
Other	Joint aspiration and fluid analysis (infection, cystals)
Imaging	Joint ultrasound
	Plain X-rays
	MRI for soft tissue evaluation (if indicated)
Treatment	Analgesia
	Anti-inflammatories (plus gastric protection)
	Steroids (if indicated)
	Mobilise within the limits of the pain / physiotherapy
	Treat the underlying cause
	Disease modifying anti-rheumatic drugs (DMARDs)
	Lifestyle modifications e.g. Weight loss
Red flags	Acute hot, swollen joint.

BACK PAIN = a general term for a common set of symptoms relating to discomfort in the back, can be moderate to severe and have a major impact on function and quality of life [7]

Onset + Duration
- When did it start / how long has it been going on for?

Acute (<6 weeks)
Subacute (6–12 weeks)
Chronic (>12 weeks)

Characterisation
- Can you describe the pain?
- Is it sharp, dull, burning or throbbing etc.

Location
- Is the pain localised or generalised?
- Is there radiation to the legs?
- Which parts of the back are affected - e.g. lumbar or thoracic etc.

Radiation to the legs is a feature of sciatica.

Severity
- How severe is the pain on a scale of 1–10?

Ask the patient to quantify the intensity of their pain and describe the impact this has on their quality of life.

Timing
- Is the pain constant or intermittent?
- Worse in the morning or at night?

Establish if there a pattern to the back pain.

Triggers
- What makes it worse (e.g. bending, lifting, rest)?
- What helps the back pain (e.g. rest, medications, warm bath)?
- What is your job?
- Do you engage in heavy physical work or prolonged sitting/standing?
- Any history of trauma or heavy lifting?
- Any recent falls or accidents?

Important to identify the exacerbating and relieving factors. Occupational history is important both to understand what it is that they do and what the back pain stops them from doing.

Associated Symptoms
- Any numbness, tingling, weakness, or bowel/bladder dysfunction?

Clarify if there might be a neurological component.

- Are you experiencing any fever, weight loss, or night sweats?

Ascertain if there is any constitutional upset.

Common Causes of Back Pain [8]

Musculo-skeletal	Traumatic damage, lumbar strain / sprain
	Degenerative disc disease, prolapsed intervertebral disc,
	Spondylolithesis, facet joint arthritis
Neurological	Sciatica, spinal stenosis, cauda equina syndrome
Inflammatory	Ankylosing spondylitis, rheumatoid arthritis
Infectious	Vertebral osteomyelitis, discitis, epidural abscess
Cancer	Metastatic deposits, multiple myeloma
Referred pain	Pancreatitis, renal tract stones, AAA, PID.

Approach to Management

A comprehensive approach helps in the proper evaluation, diagnosis, and management of patients presenting with back pain, ensuring that serious causes are not missed while managing more common, benign conditions conservatively [9].

Blood tests	FBC, U&E's, Calcium, Phosphate
	Inflammatory markers
	Auto-immune profile e.g. Rheumatoid factor and anti-CCP AB's.
	ANA, ANCA, HLA B-27 serology
Other	Nerve conduction studies
Imaging	Plain film X-rays
	CT / MRI scanning
Treatment	Analgesia
	Anti-inflammatories (plus gastric protection)
	Steroids (if indicated)
	Mobilise within the limits of the pain / physiotherapy
	Avoid prolonged bed rest
	Treat the underlying cause
	Lifestyle modification
Red flags	<20 or > 50 years old with new-onset back pain (potential malignancy, infection)
	Changes in bowel or bladder function

FATIGUE = is a common referral into rheumatology specialist service and is characterised by extreme tiredness and individuals feeling tired all of the time [10]

Characterisation
- Can you describe what you mean by fatigue?

Getting a verbatim description 'feeling like death warmed up', 'I feel like wading through treacle' are useful characterisations as fatigue means different things to different people.

Onset + Duration
- When did the fatigue start?
- Do you feel tired all the time or does it come and go?
- Was the onset sudden or gradual?

It is useful to get an idea of the time course of fatigue and understand whether it is acute or chronic.

Pattern + Progression
- Is the fatigue worsening, improving, or staying the same?
- Is there any relief with rest or sleep?

Does the fatigue relate to specific events and precipitants and recover from rest as one might expect or is it all encompassing with no relief.

Severity + Impact
- How severe is the fatigue on a scale of 1 to 10?
- How is it affecting your daily activities (work, social life, etc.)?
- Are there specific times of day when it is worse?

Can you get a quantifiable measure of the fatigue in order to understand its impact and track changes over time.

Sleep + Rest
- How many hours do you sleep each night?
- Do you feel refreshed when you wake up?
- Do you experience difficulty falling asleep, staying asleep, or waking early?
- Do you snore or has anyone noticed periods of stopped breathing during sleep?

Sleep quantity and quality are useful indicators. If the individual is not getting high quality refreshing sleep then review their sleep hygiene and also ask about snoring (check with their partner) as they could have obstructive sleep apnoea. Poor quality sleep and poor sleep habits are signs of depression.

Associated Symptoms
- Weight loss or gain?
- Fever or night sweats?
- Changes in your skin or hair?

Constitutional upset may reveal an underlying serious condition such as a chronic indolent infection or malignancy.

- Changes in appetite or bowel habits?

Could there be a GI disorder leading to malabsorption and malnutrition.

- Do you experience any muscle or joint pains?

Rheumatological disorders can lead to muscle inflammation, weakness and fatigue.

- Any depression, anxiety, or stress?
- Are you currently experiencing significant stress at work, home, or in relationships?
- Have there been any recent life changes, such as a new job, loss of a loved one, or financial stress?
- Have you been feeling down, hopeless, or disinterested in things that normally bring you joy?

Ask specifically about mental health and life events. Is there something keeping them up at night? Is there a background history of depression for instance.

- Memory or concentration issues?
- Headaches or dizziness?

Consider neuro-psychological disorders as contributors to fatigue.

Medications + Alcohol
- Are you taking any sedatives?

Review the medication list to look for treatments that may have an effect on energy levels.

- How much have you been drinking recently?

Alcohol excess or changes in drinking patterns can lead to fatigue.

Exposure
- Have you had any recent infections, such as colds, flu, or COVID-19?

Post-viral fatigue is a recognised phenomenon so ask about the prodrome of the fatigue and occurrence of recent illnesses.

- Have you travelled recently, especially to areas where certain infections (e.g. malaria) are prevalent?

Foreign travel may provide a clue as to a potential communicable disease that could be implicated in fatigue.

Common Causes of Fatigue [11]

Endocrine	Newly diagnosed or poorly controlled Diabetes mellitus
	Hypothyroidism, Adreno-cortical insufficiency, Cushing's syndrome
	Menopause, Hypogonadism.
Haematologic	Anaemia, chronic bleeding, leukaemia, lymphoma.
Cardiac	Congestive cardiac failure, coronary artery disease / myocardial insufficiency, arrhythmias.
Respiratory	Obstructive sleep apnoea, asthma, COPD.
GI	Malabsorption e.g. Coeliac disease, IBD, pernicious anaemia,
	Chronic liver disease
Neurological	Cerebrovascular disease, multiple sclerosis, Parkinson's disease,
	Chronic fatigue syndrome.
Musculo-skeletal	Chronic pain syndromes, fibromyalgia, rheumatoid arthritis, SLE.
Psychiatric	Anxiety, stress, depression, burnout.
Infectious disease	Fatigue is common during and after infections due to immune response.
	Viral infections (e.g. mononucleosis, COVID-19, flu).
	Chronic infections (e.g. tuberculosis, HIV / AIDS).
	Persistent infections can cause ongoing fatigue.
	Post-viral fatigue. Fatigue may persist even after recovery from the initial viral illness.
Metabolic	Chronic renal disease and uraemia
	Electrolyte imbalance e.g. Hyponatraemia and hypokalaemia
	Vitamin deficiencies e.g. B12, iron, folate, vitamin D.
	Obesity - due to the additional effort required for ADL'S
Medications	Sedatives, antihistamines, beta-blockers, and certain antidepressants can cause fatigue as a side effect.
Malignancy	Both cancer itself and its treatments (chemotherapy, radiation) can cause profound fatigue.

Approach to Management

The causes of fatigue span multiple systems and require a detailed history, examination, and investigations to identify the underlying issue [12].

Blood tests	FBC, U&E's, LFT'S, TFT's
	Serum electrolytes inc calcium and magnesium
	Inflammatory markers
	Haematinics / blood film / Fe studies
	Vitamin D
	9 AM cortisol, 9 AM testosterone (if indicated)
	Fasting blood glucose / random glucose / HbA1c
	Viral serology (e.g. Epstein-Barr virus, HIV, hepatitis panel)
	Auto-immune screening (e.g. ANA, ANCA, rheumatoid factor)
Imaging	CXR
	Echocardiography (if indicated)
Other	ECG
	Epworth sleepiness scale score
	Sleep studies (polysomnography)
	Psychological screening tools (e.g. PHQ-9, GAD-7)
Treatment	Emphasis good sleep hygiene and routine
	Maintain good diet, nutrition and hydration
	Reduce or eliminate alcohol
	Relaxation techniques and self-care
	Treat the underlying abnormality
Red flags	Daytime somnolence
	Significant weight loss
	Night sweats

INTERESTING FACT: The term "orthopaedics" comes from the Greek words *orthos*, for straight and *paideion* (children). The term was first used in 1741 by French physician Nicolas Andry [13]. Orthopaedic surgeons have been friendly, helpful and holistic ever since.

References

1. Taylor PC, Van de Laar M, Laster A, et al. Call for action: incorporating wellness practices into a holistic management plan for rheumatoid arthritis—going beyond treat to target. RMD Open. 2021;7:e001959.
2. Haas R, Gorelik A, Busija L, et al. Prevalence and characteristics of musculoskeletal complaints in primary care: an analysis from the population level and analysis reporting (POLAR) database. BMC Prim Care. 2023;24:40.

3. National Academies of Sciences, Engineering, and Medicine; Health and Medicine Division; Board on Health Care Services; Committee on Identifying Disabling Medical Conditions Likely to Improve with Treatment. Selected Health Conditions and Likelihood of Improvement with Treatment. Washington (DC): National Academies Press (US). 2020. Musculoskeletal Disorders.

4. Foster NE, Hartvigsen J, Croft PR. Taking responsibility for the early assessment and treatment of patients with musculoskeletal pain: a review and critical analysis. Arthritis Res Ther. 2012;14(1):205.

5. Keenan, A.-m., Tennant, A., Fear, J., Emery, P. and Conaghan, P.G. (2006), Impact of multiple joint problems on daily living tasks in people in the community over age fifty-five. Arthritis Rheum, 55:757–64.

6. Barre A. (2024) understanding joint disorders: causes, symptoms, and treatment options. Int J Clin Rheumatol. 2024;19(3):88–91.

7. Bardin LD, King P, Maher CG. Diagnostic triage for low back pain: a practical approach for primary care. Med J Aust. 2017;206(6):268–73.

8. Hoy D, Bain C, Williams G, March L, et al. A systematic review of the global prevalence of low back pain. Arthritis Rheum. 2012;64(6):2028–37.

9. Macfarlane GJ, Beasley M, Jones EA, et al. The prevalence and management of low back pain across adulthood: results from a population-based cross-sectional study (the MUSICIAN study). Pain. 2012;153(1):27–32.

10. Latimer KM, Gunther A, Kopec M. Fatigue in adults: evaluation and management. Am Fam Physician. 2023;108(1):58–69. PMID: 37440739

11. National Institute for Health and Care Excellence. Clinical Knowledge Summary. Tiredness/fatigue in adults. 2021. https://cks.nice.org.uk/topics/tiredness-fatigue-in-adults/. Accessed 10th June 2024.

12. Cornuz J, Guessous I, Favrat B. Fatigue: a practical approach to diagnosis in primary care. Can Med Assoc J. 2006;174(6):765–7.

13. Kohler R. Nicolas Andry de bois-regard (Lyon 1658-Paris 1742): the inventor of the word "orthopaedics" and the father of parasitology. J Child Orthop. 2010 Aug;4(4):349–55.

Chapter 11
Neurology

Abstract The central and peripheral nervous system are key to our survival. The internal regulatory functions, the conscious control of movement, our sensory awareness and our ability to navigate and interact with the world are all down to a healthy, functioning set of complex neuronal circuitry. The human brain is the most complex object in the known universe, it contains 100 billion neurons and the spinal cord 13.5 million.

Multiple types of disease processes can disrupt the flow of nerve signals around the body and the majority of neurological pathologies are manifested by deficiencies or interferences of normal signalling; paralysis, sensory deficits, abnormal movements. Key to understanding the underlying aetiology of such disorders is recognising the pattern of interference, is this an upper or lower motor neurone lesion, what dermatome or spinal level is the disruption at, is there cerebellar involvement and so on. The good diagnostician is able to trace where the break in the circuitry might be and appreciate the origin based on careful history taking.

Keywords Brain · Central nervous system · Peripheral nervous system · Headache · Cerebro-vascular disease · Seizure · Epilepsy · Tremor · Paraesthesia

Introduction

Neurology is the medical field that studies the nervous system (the brain, spinal cord, nerves and the muscles they innervate), including its normal functioning, diseases, and disorders. Approximately 60% of the human brain is made of fat and weighs about 3 pounds, making it the fattiest organ in the body. The most common neurological disorders include epilepsy (a tendency to seize), stroke and Alzheimer's disease [1]. Table 11.1 outlines the common presenting complaints including headache and sensory disturbance and Table 11.2 summarises common neurological conditions that may affect the body along with their associated pattern of signs and symptoms.

P. Grant, *The Concise Guide to Medical History Taking*,
https://doi.org/10.1007/978-3-031-91474-4_11

Table 11.1 Summary table of neurology presenting complaints and differential diagnoses [2]

Neurology system presenting complaints	Commonly associated conditions
Headache	Tension headaches, cluster headaches, migraines, intracranial haemorrhage, meningitis, tumours
Seizures	Epilepsy, head trauma, brain tumours, infections (e.g. meningitis, encephalitis), metabolic imbalances, or stroke
Sensory disturbance	Peripheral neuropathies, multiple sclerosis, radiculopathies, stroke, spinal cord compression
Motor dysfunction / paralysis	Stroke, Guillain-Barré syndrome, multiple sclerosis, motor neuron disease (e.g. amyotrophic lateral sclerosis), myasthenia gravis, muscular dystrophies
Dizziness / vertigo	Vestibular dysfunction (e.g. benign paroxysmal positional vertigo, Meniere's disease), brainstem stroke, multiple sclerosis, or vestibular migraines
Cognitive impairment / confusion	Infections (e.g. encephalitis, meningitis), metabolic disorders, drug toxicity, stroke, or dementia (e.g. Alzheimer's disease)
Gait disturbances	Parkinson's disease, cerebellar ataxia, spinal cord lesions, peripheral neuropathy, normal pressure hydrocephalus
Tremor / involuntary movements	Parkinson's disease, essential tremor, Huntington's disease, medication side effects, metabolic disturbances (e.g. liver disease)
Syncope / loss of consciousness	Seizures, transient ischemic attacks (TIAs), stroke, vasovagal syncope, cardiac-related issues (e.g. arrhythmia)

Background History for the Neurological System

Understanding the patient's background and risk factors, as well as any family history is very important in neurological disorders, so before you get started it's useful to establish the following [3].

- History of previous medical or surgical problems affecting the brain or nervous system and any previous investigations such as brain scans, EEG's, procedures such as head and neck radiotherapy or neurosurgery including pituitary surgery or tumour removal?
- What are their risk factors for cerebrovascular disease; hypertension, hyperlipidaemia, diabetes, smoking, alcohol?
- Do they have a family history of any neurological conditions, (especially Alzheimer's and Huntingdon's disease as these have a genetic component)? Clarify at what ages these conditions occurred.
- Ask about their work to clarify if there is any potential occupational exposure to toxins.
- Medications—multiple drugs, both prescribed and recreational, as well as alcohol can impact the nervous system. Make sure that you get a full list of what they are taking, including narcotics.
- Constitutional upset—have you lost any weight recently? Have your diet or eating patterns changed?

Table 11.2 Summary table of common Neurological conditions and associated symptoms [1]

Common Neurology conditions	Common symptoms
Migraine	Unilateral headaches ('hemi-cranium'), nausea and vomiting, photosensitivity, aura, neck pain and stiffness, dizziness
Epilepsy	Seizures (epilepsy = a tendency to seize), generalised or focal, aura, post-ictal confusion, incontinence
Bell's palsy	Sudden, unilateral facial weakness or paralysis, inability to close one eye, loss of taste (anterior two thirds of the tongue), hyperacusis, dry eye or excessive lacrimation on affected side
Parkinson's disease	Tremor, bradykinesia, rigidity, shuffling gait, postural instability, cognitive decline, sleep disturbance, bowel and bladder problems
Guillain-Barre syndrome	Ascending muscle weakness, areflexia, parasthesiae, difficulty walking or climbing stairs, difficulty breathing
Multiple sclerosis	Visual disturbance, diplopia, fatigue, parasthesiae, muscle weakness or spasms, difficulty walking, loss of coordination, neuropathic pain, bowel and bladder problems
Normal pressure hydrocephalus	Gait disturbances, urinary incontinence, cognitive decline
Idiopathic intracranial hypertension	Headache (worse in the morning or with straining), visual disturbances, nausea and vomiting, pulsatile tinnitus
Stroke	Sudden unilateral weakness or sensory disturbance, dysarthria / dysphasia, facial droop, loss of balance / coordination, confusion
Meningitis	Headache, neck stiffness, photophobia, pyrexia, nausea and vomiting, altered mental status, rash, seizures
Space-occupying lesion	Headache, seizures, nausea and vomiting, focal neurological deficits / mass effects, cognitive / personality changes, balance and coordination problems, papilloedema

HEADACHE = pain or discomfort in the head or face [4]

Character
- How would you best describe your headache?
- Is the pain throbbing, sharp, dull or pressure-like?

Onset + Duration
- When did it start / how long has it been going on for?
- Did the headache come on suddenly or gradually?
- Is it a single episode or recurrent?

To understand if this is a potential intracranial bleed, the speed of onset and intensity of the headache is important to establish.

Location
- Whereabouts is your headache?
- Can you point to where you are getting the pain?
- Is it superficial or deep?

A unilateral headache is more suggestive of migraine, tension headache is more frontal and bilateral can be linked to more generalised conditions. Temporal arteritis pain is more superficial.

- Does the pain spread anywhere?

Clarify if the pain radiates e.g. to the neck, face or eyes.

Severity
- On a scale of 1–10, how severe is the headache?
- Has it affected your daily activities or work?

The greater the severity and the impact the more sinister the likely pathology.

Precipitants
- What sets the headache off?
- Is it worse in the morning or with certain activities?

Assess if the headache is linked to stress, certain foods, physical activity, exertion, coughing, straining etc. Raised intracranial pressure headaches are normally worse in the mornings.

- What helps improve the headache?
- Do any of the following help; rest, medication, darkness etc.?
- Any recent head injury or trauma?

A preceding head injury may slowly or quickly evolve.

- Are you experiencing any recent stress or major life events?

Stress and life events can definitely exacerbate headaches.

Associated symptoms
- Do you experience nausea or vomiting?
- Any sensitivity to light or sound?
- Do you have neck stiffness?
- Features of meningeal irritation.
- Any visual disturbances? For example, blurred vision, double vision, visual aura.
- Do you feel dizzy or off-balance?

Could be impacting on cerebellar or inner ear function.

- Any fever or confusion?

Assess potential for an underlying infection.

- Have you noticed any weakness, numbness, or difficulty speaking?

Look for neurological / motor deficits.

Common Causes of Headaches [5]

Neurological	Migraines, tension headache, cluster headaches, trigeminal neuralgia, idiopathic intracranial hypertension, space-occupying lesions, hydrocephalus, optic neuritis
Vascular	Sub-arachnoid haemorrhage, intracranial haemorrhage, temporal arteritis, cerebro-vascular accident (stroke/TIA). Hypertension.
Infections	Meningitis, Encephalitis, Sinusitis
Ophthalmological	Glaucoma, eye strain, misalignment, uveitis, scleritis
Medication	Medication overuse headache, nitrates, SSRI's
Psychological	Stress, anxiety, teeth grinding

Approach to Management

Full neurological examination is important to assess for focal neurological deficits and signs of raised intracranial pressure such as papilloedema. Check baseline observations such as blood pressure [6].

Blood tests	FBC, U&E's, LFT's
	Inflammatory markers
Other	Lumbar puncture; cells, glucose, protein etc
Imaging	**CT Head (non-contrast):** for acute headache with suspected haemorrhage or trauma
	MRI Brain: for evaluation of tumours, demyelination (multiple sclerosis), or structural lesions
	CT or MR Angiography: for suspected aneurysm, arteriovenous malformation, or vasculitis
Treatment	Analgesia
	Remove any precipitants
	Treat the underlying cause
	Lifestyle modifications
Red flags	Thunderclap headaches
	Meningism
	Altered level of consciousness
	Focal neurological deficits
	Features of raised intracranial pressure

SEIZURES = a sudden, uncontrolled burst of electrical activity in the brain, causing abnormal movements, behaviour, sensations and changes in level of consciousness. Also known as a 'fit'. The term 'epilepsy' simply means a 'tendency to seize' and relates to the fact that we all have a different seizure threshold [7]

Characterisation
- What do you mean by a seizure?
- Can you describe what happens when you have a fit or seizure?
- Was there any loss of consciousness?

An eyewitness is usually required to establish key features; generalised or focal onset, tonic-clonic movements, stiffening, jerking, loss of awareness, staring spells etc.

Onset + duration
- When did it start / how long has it been going on for?
- How long did the seizure last for?
- Is this the first episode.
- If not, was it the same as previous seizures.
- How long did it go on for?

Prodrome
- Can you describe what happened before you had the seizure?
- How were you feeling?
- What were you doing?

Clarify what activity was the patient involved in - were they sleep deprived, stressed or agitated. Did the patient experience any warning signs such as an aura (visual, auditory, olfactory sensations, deja vu).

Post-ictal
- What happened after the seizure?
- How long were you / the patient unconsciousness for?
- Was there any confusion, fatigue, muscle soreness after the seizure? How long did it take before you felt back to normal?

Clarify the details of the post-ictal phase.

Associated Symptoms
- Was there any tongue biting, incontinence, or injuries during the seizure?

These are all common features associated with uncontrolled seizure activity.

Precipitants
- Any new medications recently?
- Any alcohol or recreational drug use?

Alcohol excess, withdrawal, narcotics and many medications can predispose to seizures.

- Any recent illnesses, high temperatures or infections?

Intercurrent illness can tip an individual over the seizure threshold.

- Have you been under much stress recently or been sleep deprived?
- Any recent head trauma?

Traumatic brain injury can cause swelling and cerebral irritation.

- Flashing lights / sensitive to strong lights?

Photosensitive epilepsy (warning thereof) is something familiar to all PlayStation owners.

Common Causes of Seizures [8]

Neurological	Epilepsy, head trauma, stroke, space occupying lesions
Infections	Meningitis, encephalitis, brain abscess, sepsis
Metabolic	Hypoglycaemia, hyponatraemia, hypocalcaemia, uraemia, hepatic encephalopathy
Toxins	Alcohol, drugs e.g. Cocaine, amphetamines, benzodiazepenes, anti-depressants, anti-psychotics
Cardiovascular	Arrhythmias giving rise to syncope. Poor perfusion leading to cerebral hypoxia
Psychological	Stress, pseudoseizures, Munchausen's

Approach to Management

Seizures can be caused by a wide range of neurological, metabolic, and systemic conditions. A detailed history, targeted investigations, and appropriate management are crucial for treating the underlying cause and preventing further episodes [9]. Red flags, such as prolonged seizures, sudden-onset seizures in adults, or seizures with associated neurological deficits, warrant urgent evaluation.

Blood tests	FBC, U&E's, LFT's
	Inflammatory markers
	Toxicology screen
Imaging	**CT scan:** Initial imaging in acute settings to rule out stroke, haemorrhage, or brain tumour
	MRI scan: Provides more detailed imaging, especially for structural abnormalities, tumours, and evidence of previous stroke or scarring
Other	**Electroencephalogram (EEG):** to detect abnormal electrical activity in the brain, helpful for diagnosing epilepsy or non-epileptic events (e.g. psychogenic seizures)
	Lumbar puncture (if indicated)
	ECG
Treatment	ABCDE
	Anticonvulsant medication if prolonged seizure
	Avoidance of precipitants / seizure precautions
	Treat the underlying cause
	Prophylactic anti-convulsant medication
	Caregiver / family support
Red flags	Prolonged seizures > 5 min (status epilepticus)
	Sudden onset focal neurological deficits
	Features of meningism
	Seizure following head trauma

SENSORY DISTURBANCE = may present as reduced or increased sensation. Any condition that makes it difficult for the brain to receive, process and respond to information from the senses [10]

Onset + Duration
- When did it start / how long has it been going on for?
- Was the onset sudden or gradual?
- Has the sensory disturbance progressed or remained stable?

The pattern of timing can provide clues, sudden onset suggests a vascular underlying cause.

Characteristics
- Can you describe the sensation? Is there any loss of sensation or altered sensation?
- Do you feel abnormal sensations?
- Is there weakness associated with the sensory disturbance?

What does it feel like for the individual —numbness, tingling, burning, pins and needles, pain, or is it a heightened sense of sensation—hypersensitivity—or allodynia.

Locations
- Whereabouts is the sensory disturbance located?
- Is it unilateral or bilateral?
- Does it follow a specific pattern or distribution?

Establish whether is affects the hands, feet, face, entire limbs, whole body etc.
Is there a particular distribution e.g. glove-and-stocking distribution, dermatomal etc.

Triggers
- Do certain positions or activities trigger or relieve the symptoms?

What brings it on. Certain stress positions that stretch nerves may be the root cause e.g. sciatica.

- Is there anything that worsens or alleviates the symptoms?
- Are you taking any medications that might cause sensory disturbance?
- Have you been exposed to any toxins?

For example, chemotherapeutic agents, certain antibiotics like metronidazole, antiviral agents, alcohol, heavy metals.

Associated Symptoms
- Do you have any motor symptoms, such as weakness or difficulty moving?

Alongside the sensory disturbance characterise any motor deficits.

- Any issues with balance or coordination?

Consider whether there could alsobe cerebellar involvement?

- Do you have problems with vision or double vision?

Is there optic neuritis or a cranial nerve palsy caused by mass effect.

- Any recent bladder or bowel dysfunction?

Is there autonomic nervous system involvement or loss of sensation to certain body parts?

- Fever, weight loss, or other systemic symptoms?

Common Causes of Sensory Disturbances [11]

Neurological	Stroke, Multiple sclerosis, space occupying lesions, spinal cord
	Compression, carpal tunnel syndrome, Guillain-Barre syndrome
Metabolic	Diabetes mellitus, hypo / hypercalcaemia, vitamin B12 deficiency
	Hypothyroidism
Toxins	Alcohol
	Heavy metals e.g. Lead
	Medications e.g. Isoniazid, Metronidazole, chemotherapy
Trauma	Nerve damage / compression
Infections	Herpes zoster, HIV neuropathy, Lyme disease

Approach to Management

Sensory disturbances can arise from a wide range of causes, from metabolic disorders and infections to serious central nervous system conditions. On examination, map out the pattern, extent of the sensory disturbance and don't forget to make sure that the patient keeps their eyes closed to make it objective [12].

Blood tests	FBC, U&E's, Calcium, TFT's, Vitamin B12
	Blood glucose levels
	Autoimmune markers e.g. ANA, rheumatoid factor
	Inflammatory markers
	Infectious disease serology (where indicated)
Other	Lumbar puncture for CSF analysis
	Nerve conduction studies +/− EMG
Imaging	MRI / CT scanning of the brain and spinal cord
Treatment	Treat the underlying condition
	Analgesia / symptomatic relief for disturbed sensation e.g. Neuropathic pain agents
Red flags	Sudden onset
	Associated motor weakness
	History of cancer
	Features of sepsis
	Bowel or bladder dysfunction (indicates spinal cord compression)

MOTOR DYSFUNCTION = a range of abnormal motor symptoms that can occur in neurological conditions, including complete paralysis and excessive muscle activity such as rigidity, tremor and gait disturbances [13]

Characterisation
- Can you describe what the actual problem is and how it is affecting you?
- Are other areas of the body involved now that weren't at first?

If the patient is describing weakness, which body parts does it affect, is it symmetrical and what does it stop / limit the person from doing.

Onset + Duration
- When did the weakness or motor abnormality start?
- Was the onset sudden or gradual?
- Has it been getting worse, improving, or fluctuating?

Clarify the pattern of dysfunction e.g. stepwise changes, relapsing and remitting, or a sudden decline.

Tremor
- Have you noticed a tremor?
- When does the tremor occur?
- Does the tremor improve with alcohol?

Resting tremor—common in Parkinson's disease
Action / intention tremor—gets worse as you get close to target.
Essential tremor—idiopathic, often familial.
Dystonic tremor—medications e.g. anti-psychotics, Wilson's disease, Huntingdon's.

Gait
- Have you had any difficulty with walking or noticed changes in the way that you walk?

A shuffling gait occurs with Parkinsonism.
Antalgic gait occurs with pain.
Spastic gait—with hemiplegia.
Neuropathic gait—high stepping due to diminished sensation.
Waddling gait—muscular dystrophy.
Ataxic gait - cerebellar issues.
Wide based gait - normal pressure hydrocephalus.

Cerebellar signs
- Any problems with coordination?

Remember the acronym DANISH
Dysdiadokinesis
Ataxia
Nystagmus

Ipsilateral tremor
Slurred speech
Hypotonia

Autonomic Dysfunction

- Do you experience any of the following;

    - Racing heartbeat at rest
    - Dizziness on standing
    - Sweating excessively or when eating
    - Difficulty adapting to low or bright light conditions
    - Foul smelling burps

Resting tachycardia, orthostatic hypotension, gustatory sweating, eye adaptation problems and offensive eructation are all symptoms of ANS dysfunction.

Associated Symptoms

- Have you noticed any sensory symptoms such as numbness or tingling?

See section above.

- Have you noticed any muscle stiffness or feeling rigid?

Causes of spasticity include, brain or spinal cord injuries, cerebral palsy, nerve degeneration, MS, stroke and CNS infections.

- Any problems with fatigue or exercise intolerance?

Features of motor weakness.

- What is your level of baseline functioning / what can you normally manage to do for yourself?

Understanding the impact on function and activities of daily living is very important in neurology history taking.

Common Causes of Motor Dysfunction [14]

Neurological	Stroke, Multiple sclerosis, spinal cord injury, cerebral palsy, peripheral neuropathy, Guillain-Barre syndrome, Myasthenia Gravis, Motor neurone disease, Parkinson's disease,
Muscular	Muscular dystrophies, Poliomyositis / Dermatomyositis
Vascular	Peripheral arterial disease, Vasculitides
Endocrine	Hypothyroidism, Cushing's syndrome, diabetes mellitus
Metabolic	Vitamin B12 deficiency, hepatic encephalopathy, Wilson's disease
Drugs	Anti-dopaminergic agents, anti-depressants e.g. SSRI's, chemotherapy agents, anticonvulsants, neuropathic pain agents e.g. Gabapentin
	Alcohol

Approach to Management

Motor dysfunction and movement disorders have a broad differential diagnosis and require a comprehensive history, examination, and targeted investigations. Management depends on the underlying cause, often requiring multidisciplinary approaches [15].

Blood tests	FBC, U&E's, LFT's, TFT's, Vitamin B12
	Inflammatory markers, Creatine kinase
	Auto-antibody screen
Other	Lumbar puncture
	Nerve conduction studies / EMG
	EEG
Imaging	CT / MRI scan brain and spinal cord
Treatment	Supportive measures
	Physiotherapy, OT and SALT review
	Treat the underlying cause where possible
	Secondary prevention in the context of cerebro-vascular disease
Red flags	Sudden onset motor weakness / rapid progression
	New onset seizures
	Bowel or bladder dysfunction

SYNCOPE = commonly known as fainting or passing out, is a loss of consciousness or blackout, often due to a temporary decrease in blood flow to the brain [16]

Onset + Duration
- What were you doing when the episode occurred?

Activity at the time of syncope can indicate the cause e.g. standing, exercising, postural changes.

- How long did you lose consciousness for?

Short duration suggests benign causes like vasovagal syncope, while prolonged unconsciousness may indicate a seizure or serious cardiac issue.

Prodrome
- Did you have any warning signs before you passed out?

Palpitations, dizziness, nausea, blurred vision, or sweating before syncope might suggest certain causes e.g. vasovagal or arrythmias.

- Did you experience chest pain or shortness of breath?

Could suggest cardiac causes like myocardial infarction or pulmonary embolism.

- Were there any neurological symptoms? For example weakness, speech difficulties, or vision changes?

May indicate a transient ischemic attack (TIA) or stroke.

Post blackout
- How did you feel after regaining consciousness?
- How long did it take before you felt back to normal again?

Confusion or prolonged recovery might suggest a seizure, while a rapid recovery is more typical of vasovagal or orthostatic syncope.

- Was there any trauma or injury from the fall?

Falls without warning could indicate a more serious cause like arrhythmia.

- Did you lose control of your bowels or bladder?
- Did you bite your tongue?

More consistent with seizures rather than straight syncope.

- Do you have a history of seizures?

Important to differentiate syncope from seizure activity.

Medications
- Any new prescriptions or changes to your medications recently?

Medications like beta-blockers, diuretics, antihypertensives, or antiarrhythmics can cause hypotension or bradycardia leading to syncope.

- Do you use alcohol or drugs?

Alcohol can induce syncope, and illicit drugs can lead to arrhythmias.

Family History
- Is there a family history of sudden death or heart disease?

Suggests inherited cardiac conditions like Long QT syndrome or hypertrophic cardiomyopathy.

Common Causes of Loss of Consciousness [17]

Neurological	Seizures, Stroke/TIA, Subarachnoid haemorrhage
Cardiovascular	Arrhythmias, structural heart disease e.g. Aortic stenosis or HOCM, acute coronary syndromes, pulmonary embolism, postural hypotension, vasovagal syncope.
Metabolic	Hypoglycaemia, electrolyte imbalances e.g. Hypokalaemia, hyponatraemia.
Medication	Anti-hypertensives, beta blockers, alcohol, drug intoxication.
Psychological	Panic attacks, hyperventilation, conversion disorder, Munchausen's

Approach to Management

Syncope is a common clinical presentation with various underlying causes ranging from benign to life-threatening. Management is based on the underlying cause, and attention to red flags can help guide urgent interventions for serious conditions [18].

Blood tests	FBC, U&E's, LFT's, TFT's
	Blood glucose and HbA1c
	Cardiac biomarkers
Other	ECG
	Ambulatory ECG / event recorder
	Tilt-table test
	Exercise stress test
	EEG
Imaging	Echocardiogram
	CT / MRI brain
	Carotid doppler ultrasound

(continued)

Treatment	Avoid precipitants
	Lifestyle modifications
	Medication management
	Treat the underlying cause
Red flags	Haemodynamic instability
	Syncope on exertion
	Family history of sudden cardiac death
	Focal neurological deficits

DIZZINESS / VERTIGO = a sensation of dizziness often relates to feeling weak, lightheaded, or woozy. Vertigo is specifically the sensation of the room spinning. There is often overlap in meaning between the two so a careful history helps to differentiate [19]

Characterisation
- Can you describe specifically what you mean by feeling dizzy or having vertigo?
- For example, spinning, light-headedness, imbalance, or faintness etc.
- Is it true vertigo (spinning or rotational sensation) or dizziness (general disorientation)?

Often you will have to help the patient distinguish between the two.

Onset + duration
- When did it start / how long has it been going on for?
- How often does it occur?
- Is it progressively getting worse?

The time frame and progression will help provide useful information.

- How long do the episodes last?
- Does the sensation go on for seconds, minutes, hours, continuous?

Precipitants
- Does anything bring on the episodes?
- Are the symptoms positional?
- Does closing your eyes help to alleviate the symptoms?

Is there a trigger or worsening with head movements or changes in posture?

- Have you experienced any recent head trauma?

Consider concussion or intracerebral bleeds.

- Have you taken any new medications recently?

Ask about antihypertensives, diuretics, ototoxic medications e.g. Gentamicin.

Associated Symptoms
- Do you experience nausea or vomiting?

Potential features of raised intracranial pressure.

- Do you have any hearing loss or ringing in the ears?
- Any recent ear infections or discharge?

Potential features of an inner ear disorder.

- Do you experience double vision or blurred vision?

Clues to intracranial pathology.

- Any difficulty walking, clumsiness, or falls?
- Any numbness, weakness, or difficulty speaking?
- Do you have chest pain, palpitations, or shortness of breath?

Suggestive of cardiovascular disease and arrythmias.

Common Causes of Dizziness / Vertigo [20]

Neurological	**Benign Paroxysmal Positional Vertigo (BPPV):** brief episodes of vertigo triggered by head movements
	Vestibular neuritis: Inflammation of the vestibular nerve, causing sudden, intense vertigo
	Meniere's disease: Vertigo, hearing loss, and tinnitus, often with aural fullness
	Migraine-associated vertigo: Vertigo occurring with or without headache in people with a history of migraines
	Stroke or transient ischemic attack (TIA): Sudden onset of vertigo with other neurological symptoms (e.g. weakness, numbness, speech difficulty)
	Multiple sclerosis: May cause dizziness or vertigo as part of broader neurological deficits
Cardiovascular	Orthostatic hypotension, vasovagal syncope
	Arrythmias, aortic stenosis
Ear / Vestibular	**Labyrinthitis:** Inflammation of the inner ear, causing vertigo and often hearing loss
	Acoustic neuroma: a benign tumour on the vestibulocochlear nerve, causing vertigo, hearing loss, and tinnitus
	Cholesteatoma: Abnormal skin growth in the middle ear that can cause vertigo and hearing loss
Metabolic	Hypoglycaemia, anaemia, thyroid disorders
Psychological	Stress, anxiety, panic, somatisation
Medication	Ototoxic drugs e.g. aminoglycosides, diuretics, chemotherapy agents anti-hypertensives, sedatives, anti-depressants

Approach to Management

A structured approach to history, examination, and investigation can help differentiate between benign and serious causes of dizziness and vertigo, guiding the appropriate management and referral to ENT, Neurology or the appropriate speciality [21]. Check for nystagmus, cranial nerve function, motor and sensory deficits, and coordination tests etc.

Blood tests	FBC, U&E's, LFT's, TFT's
	Blood glucose and HbA1c
	Inflammatory markers
Other	Audiometry
	ECG
	Ambulatory ECG (if indicated)
Imaging	CT / MRI brain scan
	MRA or carotid doppler ultrasound
	Echocardiography (if indicated)
Treatment	Symptomatic support
	Treat the underlying cause
	Consider vestibular rehabilitation if indicated
Red flags	Sudden onset severe vertigo
	Focal neurological symptoms
	Meningism

COGNITIVE IMPAIRMENT = confusion, change in mental state, memory problems, ability to think, use judgement and make decisions [22]

Characterisation
- Can you describe what problems you've been having with your thinking and memory recently?

Start with a general description of what they have been experiencing before you get into any specifics.

- Are you experiencing any of the following; agitation, aggression, hallucinations, delusions, wandering?

Features of hyperactive delirium.

- Or alternatively any of; sleepiness, lethargy, slowing down, poor attention?

Features of hypoactive delirium.

Onset + Duration
- When did it start / how long has it been going on for?
- Has it been intermittent, worsening, or stable?

A collateral history may be most useful here to get an objective assessment.
Is this an acute state (delirium) or chronic (dementia). Is the confusion constant or does it fluctuate? Clarify if the confusion is worse at certain times of the day.

Precipitants
- Have there been any recent problems with your health? For example, infections, trauma, dehydration, medication changes e.g. sedatives, opioids, anticholinergics.
- Any accompanying fever, headache, vision changes, seizures, or weakness?
- Any recent falls or head injuries?

Sub-dural haematomas can slowly increase pressure on the brain and present with confusion.

- Any changes in alcohol intake or drug use recently?

Consider intoxication or withdrawal.

- Any changes in your home / living environment or any major life events?

Situational changes can be disorientating for susceptible individuals.

Memory
- Are there problems with short-term or long-term memory?

Asking specifically about each of these aspects of cognitive performance helps to narrow down the potential structures and systems that are affected and are a useful measure of global performance.

Concentration
- Do you have difficulty focusing on tasks or conversations?

Communication
- Do you have any problems with speaking or understanding?

Decision-making
- Have you had any problems with making decisions or poor judgement?

Orientation
- Do you know whereabouts you are right now?
- Do you who know who I am?
- Do you know what time it is?

Are they oriented to time, place and person.

Abbreviated Mental Test (AMT-10)

Allocate 1 point for a correct answer, 0 for an incorrect answer.

1. What is your age?
2. What is the time (to the nearest hour)?
3. I'm going to ask you to remember an address and then ask you about it later.

   Can you remember the following '42 West Street'?

4. What is the current year?
5. What is you home address?
6. What is my job? What is this object? (show the patient a simple object)
7. What is your date of birth?
8. What year did the first world war start?
9. Who is the current Prime Minister (or equivalent)?
10. Please can you count backwards down from 20 to 1?
11. Can you recall the address I asked you to remember?

This is a screening tool only [23].

A total score of 10 is normal / no confusion.
A score < 7 suggests that cognitive impairment may be present.
4–6 moderate impairment.
< 3 severe cognitive impairment.

Common Causes of Cognitive Impairment [24]

Neurological	Cerebrovascular disease, Dementia (Alzheimer's, Lewy-body, Fronto-temporal), Traumatic brain injury Post-ictal Space-occupying lesions
Infections	Systemic infections, sepsis, UTI'S.
	CNS infections; meningitis, encephalitis
Metabolic	Hypo / hyper - glycaemia, electrolyte imbalances e.g. Hypercalcaemia, hyponatraemia, thyroid disorders, liver failure, renal failure (uraemia), vitamin B12 and / or thiamine deficiency
Cardiovascular	Hypoxia, reduced cerebral perfusion, hypertensive encephalopathy, vasculitides
Psychiatric	Psychosis, depression, anxiety, mania, sleep deprivation
Medication	Drug intoxication, alcohol excess / withdrawal, heavy metals, CO

Approach to Management

Confusion and cognitive impairment are non-specific symptoms that can be caused by a wide variety of conditions affecting the brain and other systems. A stepwise screening approach to investigations is necessary to rule out the possible causes [25]. Immediate attention to red flags and urgent management of life-threatening conditions is critical for preventing irreversible damage.

Blood tests	FBC, U&E's, LFT's, TFT's, Calcium
	Haematinics
	Blood glucose
	Inflammatory markers
	Toxicology screen
	Arterial blood gas
Other	Urinalysis
	Lumbar puncture (if indicated)
	EEG (if seizures suspected)
Imaging	CT / MRI brain scan
	CXR
Treatment	Supportive management
	Reduce potential precipitants / environmental stimuli
	Treat the underlying cause
Red flags	Sudden onset
	Focal neurological deficits
	Meningism
	Reduced level of consciousness
	New onset seizures

INTERESTING FACT: In 1817, Dr. James Parkinson published 'An Essay on the Shaking Palsy', which described "paralysis agitans" a condition that would later be renamed Parkinson's disease [26].

References

1. GBD. Neurology collaborators. Global, regional, and national burden of neurological disorders, 1990–2016: a systematic analysis for the Global Burden of Disease Study 2016. Lancet Neurol. 2019;18(5):459–80.
2. MacDonald BK, Cockerell OC, Sander JWAS, Shorvon SD. The incidence and lifetime prevalence of neurological disorders in a prospective community-based study in the UK. Brain. 2000;123(4):665–76.
3. Rees R, Moodley K. Taking a neurological history. Medicine. 2023;51(8):527–30.
4. Levin M. Classification and diagnosis of primary headache disorders. Semin Neurol. 2022;42(4):406–17.
5. Olesen J. The international classification of headache disorders: history and future perspectives. Cephalalgia. 2024;44(1):3331024231214731.
6. Giamberardino MA, Affaitati G, Costantini R, Guglielmetti M, Martelletti P. Acute headache management in emergency department. A Narrative Rev Intern Emerg Med. 2020 Jan;15(1):109–17.
7. Berg AT, Berkovic SF, Brodie MJ, et al. Revised terminology and concepts for organisation of seizures and epilepsies: report of the ILAE commission on classification and terminology, 2005-2009. Epilepsia. 2010;51:676–85.
8. National Institute of Neurological Disorders and Stroke. Epilepsy and Seizures. 2025. https://www.ninds.nih.gov/health-information/disorders/epilepsy-and-seizures
9. National Institute for Health and Care Excellence. Clinical knowledge summary. Managing an epileptic seizure. 2024. https://cks.nice.org.uk/topics/epilepsy/management/managing-an-epileptic-seizure/
10. Douglass C, McDermott CJ. Assessment and diagnosis of sensory disturbance. InnovAiT. 2009;2(9):531–7.
11. Bass C. Conversion and dissociation syndromes. In: Schapira AV, et al., editors. Neurology and Clinical Neuroscience. Mosby; 2007. p. 249–57. ISBN 9780323033541.
12. Abhinav K, Edwards R, Whone A. Numbness and sensory disturbance. In: Abhinav K, Edwards R, Whone A, editors. Rapid neurology and neurosurgery; 2018.
13. Teixeira AL. Introduction to the movement disorders: definition and clinical phenotypes. In: Teixeira A, Stimming EF, Ondo WG, editors. Movement disorders in psychiatry. New York: Oxford University Press; 2022.
14. Selwa LM, Gelb DJ. Movement disorders. In: Introduction to clinical neurology. 4th ed. Oxford Academic; 2013.
15. Mahoney CJ, Sleeman R, Errington W. Assessment of suspected motor neuron disease. BMJ. 2022;379:e073857.
16. Brignole, M. Moya, A. de Lange, F. 2018 ESC guidelines for the diagnosis and management of syncope, Eur Heart J, Volume 39, Issue 21, 01 June 2018, Pages 1883–1948.
17. Kenny R, Bhangu J, King-Kallimanis B. Epidemiology of syncope/collapse in younger and older Western patient populations. Prog Cardiovasc Dis. 2013;55(4):357–63.
18. NICE. Transient loss of consciousness ('blackouts') in over 16s (quality standard). National Institute for Health and Care Excellence; 2022. http://www.nice.org.uk
19. BMJ Best Practice. Overview of Vertigo. 2024. https://bestpractice.bmj.com/topics/en-gb/965
20. Post RE, Dickerson LM. Dizziness: a diagnostic approach. Am Fam Physician. 2010;82(4):361–8. 369

21. Dommaraju S, Perera E. An approach to vertigo in general practice. Aust Fam Physician. 2016;45:4.
22. Roy E. Cognitive Impairment. In: Gellman MD, Turner JR, editors. Encyclopedia of behavioral medicine. New York: Springer; 2013.
23. Hodkinson HM. Evaluation of a mental test score for assessment of mental impairment in the elderly. Age Ageing. 1972;1(4):233–8.
24. Knopman DS. Cognitive impairment and other dementias. In: Goldman L, Schafer AI, editors. *Goldman-Cecil medicine*. 26th ed. Philadelphia, PA: Elsevier; 2020. 2020:chap 374.
25. Galvin, J. Sadowsky, C (2012) Practical guidelines for the recognition and diagnosis of dementia. J Am Board Fam Med 25(3), 367–382.
26. Parkinson J. An essay on the shaking palsy. London: Sherwood, Neely and Jones; 1817.

Chapter 12
Ophthalmology

Abstract Ophthalmology is the study and treatment of eye related diseases. The brain is the only organ in our bodies more complex than the eye and there are over one million nerves connecting each eye to the brain.

A good history is of paramount importance, and it is critical to take a careful account of a patient's eye symptoms. Additionally, it can help you to understand the impact of the condition on the individual and identify any obstacles to treatment. Visual abilities may deteriorate with age and fall into the categories of decreased distance vision and reduced near sight vision. In the acute setting we may see more along the lines of patients with red, sore, painful eyes, or other specific eye symptoms such as double vision, eyelid swelling, excessive lacrimation or increased sensitivity to light amongst others. Interestingly there are no pain receptors inside the eye itself, so an individual may have a serious condition such as glaucoma or macular degeneration and not be aware of this until permanent eye damage has occurred.

Keywords Double vision · Ophthalmoplegia · Hemianopia · Optic neuritis · Glaucoma · Retinopathy · Cataracts · Acute red eye · Photophobia

Introduction

Ophthalmic conditions such as conjunctivitis and cataracts are very common, as well as neurological issues which can interfere with the sending and receiving of signals from the optic apparatus leading to visual disturbance. Many eye conditions are silent, meaning individuals might not notice symptoms until their vision is partially impaired. This is true for potentially blinding eye diseases like glaucoma, age-related macular degeneration. Ophthalmology is both a medical and surgical speciality within medicine that deals with the diagnosis and treatment of a whole range of eye disorders. In Table 12.1 there is a summary of the varied ways in which ocular disease can present and Table 12.2 lists common eye conditions and their associated symptoms.

P. Grant, *The Concise Guide to Medical History Taking*, https://doi.org/10.1007/978-3-031-91474-4_12

Table 12.1 Summary table of presenting eye complaints and differential diagnoses [1]

Ophthalmology presenting complaints	Commonly associated conditions
Blurred vision / visual disturbance	Refractive errors e.g. Myopia (near-sightedness), hyperopia (farsightedness), astigmatism, presbyopia Cataracts, retinopathy, maculopathy, retinal detachment, optic neuritis, cerebrovascular disease
Red eye	Conjunctivitis, sub-conjunctival haemorrhage, uveitis, keratitis, acute angle-closure glaucoma
Eye pain	Corneal abrasion, uveitis, scleritis, conjunctivitis, endophthalmitis, acute angle-closure glaucoma
Photophobia	Migraine, uveitis, corneal abrasion, keratitis, meningism
Proptosis	Grave's orbitopathy, orbital cellulitis, orbital tumours, orbital trauma
Eye discharge	Conjunctivitis (bacterial, viral, allergic), blepharitis, lacrimal sac infection (dacrocystitis)
Visual field defects	Cerebrovascular disease, retinal detachment, space occupying lesions e.g. Pituitary tumour impinging on the optic chiasm, MS
Floaters and flashes	Posterior vitreous detachment (PVD), retinal detachment, uveitis, vitreous haemorrhage, migraine with aura
Diplopia	Cranial nerve palsies, myasthenia gravis, thyroid eye disease, orbital trauma, cerebrovascular disease
Sudden visual loss	Central retinal artery occlusion (CRAO), retinal detachment, optic neuritis, vitreous haemorrhage, cerebrovascular disease, acute closed angle glaucoma
Gritty eyes / foreign body sensation	Corneal foreign body, corneal abrasion, dry eye syndrome, contact lens-related irritation

Table 12.2 Summary table of common Ophthalmological conditions and associated symptoms [2]

Common Eye conditions	Common symptoms
Glaucoma	Redness, pain, blurred vision, nausea and elevated intraocular pressure
Cataracts	Gradual clouding of the lens, leading to vision blurring
Conjunctivitis	Mild pain or discomfort, often with discharge and redness
Keratitis	Often associated with contact lens use, causing redness and discomfort
Uveitis	Redness around the iris (ciliary flush) and associated pain
Retinopathy	Visual disturbances, light sensitivity, floaters, impaired night vision.
Retinal detachment	Sudden onset blurring, often with flashes or floaters.
Optic neuritis	Sudden vision loss, often in one eye, with pain on eye movement.
Thyroid eye disease	Grave's orbitopathy - proptosis / exophthalmos, diplopia.
Refractive errors	Myopia, hyperopia, astigmatism, presbyopia.
Macular degeneration	Affects central vision, commonly in older adults.

Background History for Ophthalmology

Several neurological and systemic conditions affect the eyes and a large number of medical and environmental factors can play a part, so before you get started it's useful to check the following [3].

- History of previous medical or surgical problems affecting the eyes and any previous investigations such as OCT scans, visual field assessments and any eye surgeries e.g. cataract extraction, muscle surgery, glaucoma, or retinal surgery? Recurrent eye conditions include allergic conjunctivitis, uveitis, recurrent corneal erosions and herpes simplex keratitis.
- Clarify if the patient uses prescription glasses and if these are for distance or near vision.
- History of past trauma to the eye as this can explain occurrence of conditions such as cataracts and retinal detachment.
- Do they have a family history of any ophthalmological conditions (especially glaucoma as this can be hereditary, as well as retinoblastoma)?
- Medications—multiple drugs, both prescribed and recreational, as well as smoking (which is irritant) can affect the eyes. Make sure that you get a full list of what they are taking, including any eye drops. Compliance and effectiveness of administration certainly for eye drops is important to understand.

VISUAL DISTURBANCE = a change in vision [4]

Characterisation
- What is the nature of the change in your vision?
- Does it affect one or both eyes?
- Does the visual disturbance only affect a specific area of vision?

Record whether this is bilateral or unilateral and to the same extent or not. Peripheral vs central. Ask the patient to describe what they mean and clarify if they are experiencing a deterioration in their eyesight or something else e.g. blurring, double vision, loss of vision, visual field defects.

- Are there any visual distortions?

  - straight lines becoming wavy,
  - scintillating / sparkly lights,
  - objects appearing larger or smaller than they really are.
  - any curtain like sensation or shadows in the visual fields.

Visual metamorphopsia, is a visual defect that causes objects to appear warped, wavy, or rounded. It's usually caused by macular dysfunction. Scintillating scotomas can be caused by migraine or inflammation of the optic nerve for example. A curtain like change (amaurosis fugax) may signify impending stroke).

- Are you experiencing any double vision?
- Is it in one eye or only when both eyes are open?
- Does the double vison go away if you close one eye?
- Are the images side-by-side (horizontal), one above the other (vertical), or both (oblique)?
- Do you have gaps in your fields of vision?

Diplopia can be due to involvement of the cranial nerves and extra-ocular muscles.
    Disorders of cranial nerves III and IV can cause vertical diplopia.
    Attempt to map out the defect in an individual's visual fields to identify where in the ophthalmic pathway the lesion may be e.g. bitemporal hemianopia is due to a midline lesion such as a pituitary adenoma or meningioma.

Onset + Duration
- When did it start / how long has it been going on for?
- Was the disturbance sudden or gradual in onset?
- Is it constant or intermittent?

Acute changes are more likely to be vascular in origin.

Associated Symptoms

- Have you been getting any eye pain, redness, or discharge?
  Suggestive of an infection.

- Headache?

Possibly related to migraine or tension.

- Any sensitivity to light?

Photophobia can suggest meningism, but also eye conditions, eye injuries and medications such as methotrexate.

- Any flashes of light or floaters?

Indicate retinal problems.

- Any neurological symptoms such as drooping of the eyelid, motor weakness, numbness or dizziness?

Can signify CNS or PNS disorders.

Precipitants
- Does it change with lighting conditions or time of day?

Retinopathy is associated with loss of night vision.

- Does anything make the visual disturbance worse or better?
- Any history of trauma or potential for foreign bodies to get in your eye?

Check if anything has happened to them recently and ask about occupational factors e.g. welding.

- Any recent infections?

Head and neck or nasopharyngeal infections may spread.

- Any issues with weight loss, fever, or night sweats

Suggestive of malignancy or systemic disease.

Common Causes of Visual Disturbances [5]

Ocular	Refractive errors (myopia, hyperopia, astigmatism, presbyopia), Cataracts, Glaucoma, Retinal detachment, Macular degeneration, Corneal diseases, Uveitis
Neurological	Optic neuritis, stroke, migraine with aura, multiple sclerosis, space occupying lesions, cranial nerve palsies, intracranial hypertension
Vascular	Hypertensive retinopathy, central retinal artery / vein occlusion, giant cell arteritis
Infections	Conjunctivitis, herpes zoster ophthalmicus, endophthalmitis
Metabolic	Hyperosmolar symptoms of diabetes

Approach to Management

When evaluating visual disturbances, it is essential to ask targeted questions to narrow down the underlying causes, followed by thorough examination, pupil reactions, fundoscopy and visual acuity testing [6].

Blood tests	FBC, U&E's, TFT's
	Inflammatory markers
	Glucose and HbA1c
	Auto-immune markers (if indicated)
Other	Visual field testing
Imaging	Ocular coherence tomography (OCT) (if indicated)
	CT / MRI brain (if indicated)
	Fluorescein angiography
Treatment	Treat the underlying cause
	Corrective lenses or refractive surgery
Red flags	Sudden visual loss
	Painful vision loss
	Proptosis with pain

EYE PAIN / RED EYE = spectrum of signs and symptoms relating to ocular pain and inflammation [7]

Character
- What is the problem that you are having with your eyes?
- Is it one eye or both eyes?

Clarify the nature of the ophthalmological problem.

Onset + Duration
- When did it start / how long has it been going on for?
- Did it come on suddenly or gradually?
- Is it constant or intermittent?

Time course of the eye problems can be useful to understand the pathology.

Eye Symptoms
- What type of pain are you are experiencing?
- Is it sharp, dull, burning, aching?
- Is the pain worse on movement of the eye(s)?
- Does the pain spread anywhere else?
- On a scale of 0–10, how severe is the pain, if 0 is no pain and 10 is the worst pain you've ever experienced?

Ask the patient to describe their pain.

- Is there any discharge?

Find out what is the colour and consistency.

- Are there associated symptoms such as itching, grittiness, tearing, vision changes?

Clarify any features of inflammation or infection.

Precipitants
- Does anything make the pain worse? For example, blinking, touching the eye, moving the eye, bright lights?
- Any recent eye trauma or foreign body sensations?
- What was the mechanism of injury e.g. chemical, blunt or sharp / penetrating?

Ask about the details of any eye injury or exposure to toxic agents or irritants.

- Exposure to chemicals, smoke, or infectious agents?

Any known allergies e.g. medications, environmental etc.?

- Does anything make the pain better? For example, analgesia, cool water, warm compress, removing contact lenses, dimming the lights?

Associated Symptoms
- Any headaches or photophobia?

Consider meningism and intracranial pathology.

- Are there any problems with eye or eye lid movements?

Consider cranial nerve palsies.

- Any joint pain, oral ulcers or urinary problems?

Consider autoimmune linked conditions.

Common Causes of Eye Pain / Red Eye [8]

Ocular	Conjunctivitis (bacterial, viral, allergic)
	Keratitis (corneal inflammation)
	Uveitis, Scleritis, corneal abrasions
	Acute closed angle glaucoma
Infections	Endophthalmitis (infection inside the eye)
	Herpes simplex or zoster keratitis
Neurological	Optic neuritis
Autoimmune	Rheumatoid arthritis, SLE, sarcoidosis, thyroid eye disease
Vascular	Temporal / giant cell arteritis

Approach to Management

When assessing a patient with eye pain or red eye, a detailed and structured history is crucial for identifying the underlying cause, followed by fundoscopy, slit-lamp examination and special tests [9].

Blood tests	FBC, U&E's, TFT's
	Inflammatory markers
	Auto-antibody testing
Other	Eye swabs
	Tonometry to measure eye pressure
	Visual acuity testing
	Fluorescein staining
Imaging	Ultrasound
	CT / MRI orbits
Treatment	Analgesia / symptom relief / anti-inflammatories
	Treat the underlying cause
	Clean / protect the eye(s) where necessary

(continued)

Red flags	Moderate to severe pain is a red flag symptom and requires an urgent ophthalamology review
	Sudden vision loss
	Proptosis with eye pain

INTERESTING FACT: Even though the retina detects only 3 colours, red, blue and green, we can distinguish over ten million different colours. Eyes detect 36,000 pieces of information an hour, and if each of your eyes were a digital camera, they would have 576 megapixels [10].

References

1. Mahjoub H, Ssekasanvu J, Yonekawa Y. Most common ophthalmic diagnoses in eye emergency departments: a multicenter study. Am J Ophthalmol. 2023;254:36–43.
2. Galloway NR, Moaku W, Galllowy P, Browning A. Common eye diseases and their management. 5th ed. Springer; 2022. ISBN 978-3-031-08449-2.
3. Takusewanya M. How to take a complete eye history. Community Eye Health. 2019;32(107):44–5. Epub 2019 Dec 17
4. Dandona L, Dandona R. Revision of visual impairment definitions in the international statistical classification of diseases. BMC Med. 2006;4:7.
5. Collaborators, GBD & Study, Vision. Causes of blindness and vision impairment in 2020 and trends over 30 years, and prevalence of avoidable blindness in relation to VISION 2020: the Right to Sight: an analysis for the Global Burden of Disease Study. 9;2021.
6. Pilling RF, Allen L, Bowman R, et al. Clinical assessment, investigation, diagnosis and initial management of cerebral visual impairment: a consensus practice guide. Eye. 2023;37:1958–65.
7. Dunlop A, Wells J. Approach to red eye for primary care practitioners. Prim Care. 2015;42(3):267–84.
8. Lansingh VC, Eckert KA, Ramos SV, et al. From acute disease to red flags: a review of the diverse spectrum of red eye encountered in the primary care setting. Primary Health Care. 2018;8(4)
9. Moorfields Eye Hospital. GP handbook—common eye condition management. Moorfields Eye Hospital NHS Foundation Trust; 2017. https://www.moorfields.nhs.uk/content/gp-handbook.
10. Clark R. Visual astronomy of the deep sky. Cambridge: Cambridge University Press and Sky Publishing; 1990. p. 355.

Chapter 13
Ear, Nose, and Throat

Abstract Oto-rhino-laryngology is the speciality of caring for people with ear, nose and throat problems. ENT specialists treat hearing, swallowing and speech, breathing and sleep issues, allergies, sinus disorders, and a multitude of head and neck conditions including thyroid lumps and base of skull tumours. Because these orifices are in close contact with the outside world, they are especially prone to infections and allergic responses. ENT conditions account for approximately 8% of all referrals into secondary care.

Keywords Epistaxis · Hearing loss · Vertigo · Thyroid nodule · Snoring · Obstructive sleep apnoea · Rhinorrhoea · Vertigo · Pharyngitis · Meniere's disease · Earwax impaction

Introduction

Disorders of the oral cavity, throat, nasopharynx, upper respiratory tract, the hearing apparatus, the larynx and the neck in general are very common and tend to be combined under the care of specialist ENT clinicians who can treat such conditions from hearing loss to tonsillitis and head and neck cancers, both medically and surgically. Table 13.1 outlines the common presenting complaints that an Otorhinolaryngologist would be interested in including pharyngitis and neck lumps, whereas Table 13.2 lists common ENT disorders and their associated symptoms.

Background History for the ENT System

There are multiple conditions that can affect the ears, nose and throat and it is important to establish this background, along with any relevant family history or environmental factors that can have an impact [3].

P. Grant, *The Concise Guide to Medical History Taking*, https://doi.org/10.1007/978-3-031-91474-4_13

223

Table 13.1 Summary table of ENT presenting complaints and differential diagnoses [1]

ENT presenting complaints	Commonly associated conditions
Ear pain (otalgia)	Otitis externa, otitis media, eustachian tube dysfunction, earwax impaction, TMJ disorders, mastoiditis
Hearing impairment	Conductive hearing loss; earwax impaction, otitis media with effusion, otosclerosis, choleastoma. Sensorineural hearing loss: Presbycusis, noise related damage, Meniere's disease
Tinnitus	Noise induced hearing loss, Meniere's disease, presbycusis, ototoxic medications e.g. Gentamicin, acoustic neuroma, earwax impaction
Vertigo / dizziness	BPPV, vestibular neuritis, Meniere's disease, labyrinthitis, acoustic neuroma, migraine
Nasal congestion	Allergic rhinitis (Hay fever), sinusitis (acute or chronic), viral upper respiratory infections (common cold), nasal polyps, non-allergic rhinitis
Snoring	Obstructive sleep Apnoea (OSA), obesity, enlarged tonsils / adenoids, deviated nasal septum, allergic rhinitis
Rhinorrhoea (runny nose)	Allergic rhinitis, viral upper respiratory infections, sinusitis, non-allergic rhinitis
Epistaxis (bleeding nose)	Nasal trauma, dry air, allergic rhinitis, anticoagulant medications, hypertension, hereditary haemorrhagic telangiectasia (HHT)
Anosmia (loss of smell)	Viral upper respiratory infection, chronic sinusitis, allergic rhinitis, nasal polyps, COVID-19 infection, head trauma, Klinefelter's syndrome
Pharyngitis (sore throat)	Viral pharyngitis, streptococcal pharyngitis (strep throat), tonsillitis, infectious mononucleosis, laryngopharyngeal reflux
Hoarseness (dysphonia)	Laryngitis, vocal cord nodules or polyps, recurrent laryngeal nerve palsy, gastroesophageal reflux disease, laryngeal cancer
Neck lump(s)	Lymphadenopathy, thyroid nodules / cancer, salivary gland Tumours, branchial cyst, lymphoma
Dysphagia	Tonsillitis or pharyngitis, Oesophageal stricture / malignancy, neurological disorders, achalasia

- History of previous medical or surgical problems affecting the ears, nose or throat/head and neck, such as chronic sinusitis or hearing loss, and any previous investigations such as naso-endoscopies or operations such as sinus surgery?
- History of allergies / allergens / occupational exposures / toxins / smoke / excessive noise?
- Do they have a family history of any ENT conditions / could there be a genetic component (familial adenomatous polyposis can cause nasal polyps, Usher's syndrome can can hearing loss and visual impairment, Pendred's syndrome can cause hearing impairment and thyroid problems). If there's a family history of these or similar conditions, it's important to note in the patient's medical history for further assessment and management.
- Medications—multiple drugs, both prescribed and recreational, can affect the ENT structures for example Gentamicin is well recognised to damage hearing. Make sure that you get a full list of what they are taking.

Table 13.2 Summary table of common ENT conditions and associated symptoms [2]

Common ENT conditions	Common symptoms
Otitis externa	Ear pain, ear discharge, ear canal itching, hearing loss, redness tenderness and swelling of the outer ear, fullness in the ear
Otitis media	Ear pain, hearing loss, pressure in the ear, fever, fluid drainage, irritability, balance problems
Meniere's disease	Vertigo, hearing loss, tinnitus, pressure in the ear, nausea and vomiting, balance problems
Labyrinthitis	Sudden vertigo, hearing loss, nausea and vomiting, balance problems, recent URTI symptoms
BPPV	Sudden vertigo - exacerbated by movements, nausea, balance problems, no hearing loss
Sinusitis	Nasal congestion, headache, facial pain or pressure, reduced sense of taste or smell, dental pain, fever, fatigue, post-nasal drip
Rhinitis	Runny nose, sneezing, nasal congestion, watery eyes, itchy nose or eyes, cough, fatigue, facial pressure
Obstructive sleep apnoea	Loud snoring, breathing cessation, daytime somnolence, morning headaches, poor concentration and memory, irritability, fatigue, hypertension
Tonsillitis	Sore throat, dysphagia, fever, swollen, red tonsils, cervical lymphadenopathy, halitosis, hoarse voice, fatigue
Thyroid lumps	Palpable neck swellings, dysphagia, hoarse voice, potential airway compromise, throat discomfort, features of under overactive thyroid

EAR PAIN = Otalgia. Discomfort emanating from the inner or outer ear [4]

Characterisation
- How would you describe the pain (sharp, dull, throbbing)?
- Where specifically are you getting the pain in your ear(s)?
- Any pain elsewhere e.g. in your jaw or scalp?

Ask the patient to specifically state or show where the pain is located and its nature. Consider if the pain is being referred from another structure?

Onset + Duration
- When did it start / how long has it been going on for?
- Is the pain constant or intermittent?
- Did it start suddenly or gradually?

Acute otalgia may be due to trauma or a ruptured tympanic membrane. Gradual discomfort may be due to inflammatory or infective causes.

Associated Symptoms
- Are there any other symptoms, such as hearing loss or tinnitus?

See section below

- Have you had any discharge, fever, or dizziness?

Discharge and pyrexia are suggestive of an infection, whilst dizziness suggests an inner ear involvement.

- What colour is the discharge?

Clarify if this looks clear, infective (yellow / green) or is bloody.

- Have you had any recent upper respiratory infections or ear infections?

Are they prone to infections or had a significant recent episode?

Precipitants
- Do you have any known allergies?
- Any recent changes in medications?
- Have you been exposed to loud noises, been swimming or experienced changes in altitude or pressure ie. flying or diving?

Any recent ear or head trauma? Was there a preceding injury, foreign body or environmental exposure? Is there sensitivity to a known allergen or a history of atopy? Check what they are taking including over the counter medications.

Common Causes of Ear Pain [4]

Primary otological	Eustachian tube dysfunction, trauma, barotrauma, foreign bodies, tumours (rare), glue ear, earwax build up.
Secondary	Referred pain, Temporo-mandibular joint dysfunction. Dental issues. Gastro-oesophageal reflux. Sinusitis. Sore throat.
Infections	Otitis media, otitis externa, mastoiditis

Approach to Management

Identifying and addressing potential underlying causes promptly is crucial for effective management of ear pain [5]. Otoscopic examination to check for redness, discharge, or perforation.

Blood tests	FBC, U&E's
	Inflammatory markers
Other	Audiometry
	Tympanonmetry
	Ear culture / swab / M,C & S
Imaging	CT / MRI scan
Treatment	Analgesia
	Warm compresses
	Ear toilet (if indicated)
	Treat the underlying cause
Red flags	Purulent, bloody discharge
	Systemic symptoms / features of sepsis
	Neurological symptoms

HEARING IMPAIRMENT = reduction or complete loss of ability to hear effectively. This can result from a variety of causes that span multiple systems [6]

Onset + Duration
- When did it start / how long has it been going on for?
- Was it sudden or gradual?
- Has it been getting worse over time, or does it fluctuate?

Clarify if this is a slow steady decline or has been rapidly getting worse in steps.

Characteristics
- Does the hearing impairment affect one or both ears?

Unilateral hearing loss is more likely to be conductive.

- Are there certain times or situations where it's more noticeable?

What are the environmental circumstances around the hearing impairment.

- Are there any particular types of sounds that you are struggling to hear e.g. voices, television, phone calls, high frequencies?

Associated Symptoms
- Do you ever experience any ringing in your ears?

Tinnitus is a feature of hearing loss as the nervous system tries to compensate.

- Have you experienced a fullness or pressure in your ears?

Could there be a build-up of wax or a change in pressure.

- Any history of dizziness, vertigo, nausea, or balance issues?

This is relevant to inner ear involvement.

- Do you experience pain in the ear or discharge?

See section above.

Precipitants
- Any recent ear infections or surgeries?

Inflammatory changes and infections can temporarily or permanently damage hearing.

- Any history of head trauma or noise exposure?

Check both occupational and recreational activities.

- Do you have a family history of hearing problems?

Are other family members affected and at what age of onset was their hearing loss?

- Do you have diabetes

Certain mitochondrial forms of diabetes are associated with bilateral deafness.

- Are you on any new medications?

Several medications can be ototoxic.

Common Causes of Hearing Impairment [7]

Conductive	Otitis media with effusion,
	Otosclerosis (bony overgrowth in the middle ear),
	External blockage (wax build-up, foreign body, otitis externa),
	Tympanic membrane perforation or trauma.
Sensorineural	Presbycusis (age-related hearing loss),
	Noise-induced hearing loss (prolonged loud noise exposure),
	Sudden sensorineural hearing loss (SSHL) often idiopathic or viral.
Neurological	Vestibular schwannoma (acoustic neuroma),
	Multiple sclerosis, stroke or TIA.
Infections	Viral labyrinthitis or neuritis,
	Bacterial meningitis.
Vascular	Microvascular ischaemia
Metabolic	Diabetes mellitus, hypothyroidism,
	Autoimmune inner ear disease.
Medications	Aminoglycoside antibiotics, cisplatin, loop diuretics, and high-dose salicylates (e.g. aspirin).

Approach to Management

Effective management requires a comprehensive approach that includes a detailed history, physical examination, including otoscopy to examine the ear canal and tympanic membrane for abnormalities, and often specialised investigations [8].

Blood tests	FBC, U&E's
	Inflammatory markers
	Autoimmune screen
Other	**Pure tone audiometry (PTA):** Quantifies hearing thresholds and distinguishes between conductive and sensorineural hearing loss.
	Speech audiometry: Measures ability to recognise spoken words and assess auditory discrimination.
Imaging	**MRI brain / internal auditory canals:** Especially if asymmetrical sensorineural hearing loss is present, to rule out vestibular schwannoma or other central lesions.
	CT temporal bone: Useful in suspected bony abnormalities (e.g. otosclerosis).
Treatment	Supportive management and lifestyle changes
	Hearing aids and assistive devices
	Treat the underlying cause
Red flags	Sudden, unilateral sensorineural hearing loss
	Associated neurological symptoms
	History of head trauma

VERTIGO = specifically the sensation of the room spinning [9]

Characterisation
- Can you describe specifically what you mean by having vertigo?

For example spinning, light-headedness, imbalance, or faintness etc.

- Is it true vertigo (spinning or rotational sensation) or dizziness (general disorientation)?

Often you will have to help the patient distinguish between the two.

Onset + Duration
- When did it start / how long has it been going on for?
- How often does it occur?
- Is it progressively getting worse?

The time frame and progression will help provide useful information.

- How long do the episodes last?
- Does the sensation go on for seconds, minutes, hours, continuous?

Precipitants
- Does anything bring on the episodes?
- Are the symptoms positional?
- Does closing your eyes help alleviate symptoms?

Is there a trigger or worsening with head movements or changes in posture?

- Have you experienced any recent head trauma?
- Consider concussion or intracerebral bleeds.
- Have you taken any new medications recently?

Ask about antihypertensives, diuretics, ototoxic medications e.g. gentamicin.

Associated symptoms
- Do you experience nausea or vomiting?

Potential features of raised intracranial pressure.

- Do you have any hearing loss or ringing in the ears?
- Any recent ear infections or discharge?

See sections above.

- Do you experience double vision or blurred vision?

Clues to intracranial pathology.

- Any difficulty walking, clumsiness, or falls?
- Any numbness, weakness, or difficulty speaking?
- Do you have chest pain, palpitations, or shortness of breath?

Suggestive of cardiovascular disease and arrythmias.

Common Causes of Vertigo [10]

Neurological	**Benign Paroxysmal Positional Vertigo (BPPV):** brief episodes of vertigo triggered by head movements.
	Vestibular neuritis: Inflammation of the vestibular nerve, causing sudden, intense vertigo.
	Meniere's disease: Vertigo, hearing loss, and tinnitus, often with aural fullness.
	Migraine-associated vertigo: Vertigo occurring with or without headache in people with a history of migraines.
	Stroke or transient ischemic attack (TIA): Sudden onset of vertigo with other neurological symptoms (e.g. weakness, numbness, speech difficulty).
	Multiple sclerosis: May cause dizziness or vertigo as part of broader neurological deficits.
Ear / Vestibular	**Labyrinthitis:** Inflammation of the inner ear, causing vertigo and often hearing loss.
	Acoustic neuroma: a benign tumour on the vestibulocochlear nerve, causing vertigo, hearing loss, and tinnitus.
	Cholesteatoma: Abnormal skin growth in the middle ear that can cause vertigo and hearing loss.
Psychological	Stress, anxiety, panic, somatisation.
Medication	Ototoxic drugs e.g. Aminoglycosides, diuretics, chemotherapy agents anti-hypertensives, sedatives, anti-depressants.

Approach to Management

A structured approach to history, examination, and investigation can help differentiate between benign and serious causes of vertigo, guiding the appropriate management and referral to ENT or Neurology. Check for nystagmus, cranial nerve function, motor and sensory deficits, and coordination tests etc. [11].

Blood tests	FBC, U&E's, LFT's, TFT's
	Blood glucose and HbA1c
	Inflammatory markers
Other	Audiometry
	ECG
	Ambulatory ECG (if indicated)
Imaging	CT / MRI brain scan
	MRA or carotid doppler ultrasound
Treatment	Symptomatic support
	Treat the underlying cause
	Consider vestibular rehabilitation if indicated
Red flags	Sudden onset severe vertigo
	Focal neurological symptoms
	Meningism

NASAL CONGESTION / RHINORRHOEA = a stuffy or blocked nose is a classic coryzal type symptom but can also be due to other causes. An excessively runny nose with discharge is known as rhinorrhoea and can indicate multiple local and systemic pathologies [12]

Characterisation
- What has been happening with your nose recently?
- Does it affect just one side or both?
- Is it intermittent or continuous?

Nasal congestion is common but often non-specifc manifestation of underlying nasal pathology. Details help to define the pathology.

- Have you been getting any pain in your nose?

Ask the patient to describe the type of pain and the specific nature and location.

Onset + Duration
- When did it start / how long has it been going on for?
- Did the problem develop gradually or suddenly?
- Are the symptoms constant, intermittent, or seasonal?

The time course of the nasal problem may give clues as to the underlying cause. Assess if seasons are worse at different times of the year.

Intensity
- How bothersome are the symptoms?
- Has there been any impact on daily activities or sleep?

Nasal problems can be highly irritating and potentially debilitating.

Associated Symptoms
- Are you getting any nasal discharge?
- Is the nasal discharge clear, purulent (yellow / green), or bloody?

A mucky discharge and fever is more consistent with infection and inflammation.

- Has the blockage and irritation got bad enough to cause epistaxis?
- Have you had a high temperature?
- Any sneezing, postnasal drip, or cough?

Signs of nasal irritation. Cough can be secondary.

- Any headache or facial pain?

Features of congestion and potentially sinus involvement.

Precipitants
- Have you been able to identify any specific aggravating factors, e.g. dust, pets, pollen, or irritants e.g. smoke, pollution etc.?

- Does anything improve your symptoms for exmple medications, nasal sprays, humidity, avoiding triggers? Any recent travel?
- Any close contact with people or family members who have had cold or flu-like symptoms?

Assess for allergens or environmental triggers. Relieving factors will help clarify the potential offending agent. If the individual has come in contact with unwell individuals ask about the timeframe to consider the prodrome.

Common Causes of Nasal Congestion / Rhinorrhoea [13]

Nasal	Allergic rhinitis, cold / flu, nasal polyps, deviated nasal septum, foreign bodies. Vasomotor rhinitis / non-allergic rhinitis (due to temperature, strong odours, spicy food, or environmental irritants). Enlarged adenoid tonsils
Infections	Upper respiratory tract infections, sinusitis, naso-pharyngitis.
Medications	Overuse of nasal decongestants (rhinitis medicamentosa), beta-blockers, oral contraceptive pill (hormonal changes).
Miscellaneous	Sleep apnoea, granulomatous conditions, GORD.

Approach to Management

ENT examination is useful to assess whether there is an obvious cause such as polyps. The SNOT-22 questionnaire (Sino-Nasal Outcome Test - https://www.canvasc.ca/wp-content/uploads/2021/10/SNOT22.pdf) is a detailed set of questions that can help to quantify the severity of symptoms as well as the social and emotional consequences [14].

Blood tests	FBC, U&E's
	Inflammatory markers
Other	Allergy testing, skin prick testing, specific IgE
	Naso-pharyngeal swabs for M,C & S.
Imaging	CT scan of sinuses (if indicated)
	Naso-endoscopy
	MRI scan if a tumour of complex sinus pathology suspected
Treatment	Analgesia and supportive measures e.g. humidification
	Decongestants
	Avoid triggers
	Anti-histamines
	Treat the underlying cause
Red flags	Severe or persistent headache
	Visual or neurological disturbance
	Foul-smelling discharge
	High fever

ANOSMIA = loss of smell (ability to smell, not that the patient has stopped smelling) [15]

Characterisation
- To what extent have you lost the ability to smell?
- Clarify if this is complete or partial (hyposmia) loss of smell.
- Have you noticed any changes in taste?

Taste changes often coincide with reduced smell (dysgeusia).

Onset + Duration
- When did it start / how long has it been going on for?
- Did the loss of smell start suddenly or gradually?

Note the timeframe, acute episodes of infection may be a precipitant, how soon after any recent changes did the loss of smell occur.

Associated Symptoms
- Are there any nasal symptoms like congestion, discharge, or sinus pressure?

Ascertain if there are other disorders of nasal function suggesting inflammation or infection.

- This may be a random question but have you noticed any issues with the development of sexual characteristics, fertility of erectile function? (men only)

Klinefelter's syndrome is associated with both hypogonadism and anosmia.

Precipitants
- Have you had any recent viral illnesses, like a cold, flu, or COVID-19?
- Do you have a history of nasal allergies or rhinitis?
- Have you had any recent head trauma or injury to the nose?
- Have you been exposed to toxins or chemicals, such as pesticides, solvents, or heavy smoke?
- Any new medications recently?

Establish if there are triggers that might have given rise to olfactory dysfunction through irritant or mechanical means.

Common Causes of Anosmia [16]

ENT	Allergic and non-allergic rhinitis, nasal polyps and tumours, septal deviation.
Infective	Viral URTI'S e.g. Covid-19. Chronic rhinosinusitis.
Neurological	Traumatic brain injury, neurodegenerative disease e.g. Parkinson's, Alzheimer's, Multiple Sclerosis. Space-occupying lesions.
Endocrine	Diabetes, hypothyroidism.
Genetic	Klinefelter's syndrome

Autoimmune	Sarcoidosis, Wegener's granulomatosis.
Psychological	Depression or anxiety - smell changes are reported in some psychiatric conditions. Functional neurological disorder.
Toxins	Lead, solvents, pesticides, or smoke inhalation.
	Medications; some antibiotics, antihypertensives, antiepileptics, and chemotherapy drugs.

Approach to Management

Nasal and neurological examination are good starting points [16].

Blood tests	FBC, U&E's, LFT's, TFT's
	Inflammatory markers glucose, HbA1c
	Vitamin B12 and zinc levels
Other	**Olfactory testing** - scratch-and-sniff tests to quantify the degree of smell impairment.
Imaging	**Nasal endoscopy** to visualise the nasal cavity for polyps, septal deviations, or masses.
	CT / MRI head (if indicated)
Treatment	Treat the underlying cause wherever possible.
	Olfactory training
	Lifestyle modifications
Red flags	Sudden onset severe anosmia
	Persistent unilateral anosmia
	Post trauma

SNORING = a disagreeable noise made during sleep due to airways obstruction and precipitant of divorce [17]

Characterisation
- Who has noticed that you have been snoring?
- Do you ever wake up yourself and realise that you have been snoring?
- Often the snoring is reported by others, so it is important to understand the impact on them.
- How severe is the snoring on a scale of 1 to 10?

Can they be heard through the walls and does their partner have to sleep in another room?

- Is your snoring continuous or intermittent?
- Is it present all the time.
- Has anyone observed periods where you stop breathing during sleep?

Clarify if they are having apnoeic episodes.

Onset + Duration
- When did it start / how long has it been going on for?
- Is it getting better or worse over time?

Snoring is usually present for many years before the patient (or the spouse) seeks medical attention.

Features of Snoring
- Is the snoring affected by changes in position?
- Do you snore more when sleeping on your back compared to on your side?

Has the individual tried changing sleeping positions, and did it affect their snoring.

- Do you wake up feeling rested, or do you feel fatigued?

It is common that people who snore do not experience high quality refreshing sleep.

- Do you experience daytime sleepiness or feel sleepy while driving or during other activities?

Use the Epworth Sleepiness Scale (see below) to gather more information.

- Have you noticed headaches or dry mouth upon waking?

A feature of poor nocturnal oxygenation.

- Do you experience frequent awakenings during the night?

Clarify if they wake because they are stopping breathing.

Precipitants
- Do you consume alcohol, especially close to bedtime?

Can make the individual drowsy, sluggish and unresponsive, exacerbating snoring.

- Do you use sedatives or sleep medications?
- Do you have any history of nasal congestion, allergies, or sinus problems?

All affect airflow.

- Have you been diagnosed with hypertension, heart disease, or diabetes?

All risk factors for snoring and metabolic syndrome.

The most useful way to establish the severity and impact of snoring / quantify potential obstructive sleep apnoea syndrome (OSAS) is through the use of the validated Epworth Sleepiness Scale (ESS) which produces a score from 0–24 based on the severity of symptoms - https://nasemso.org/wp-content/uploads/neuro-epworthsleepscale.pdf

Common Causes of Snoring [18]

Respiratory	Obstructive sleep apnoea (OSA), chronic nasal congestion, URTI's, nasal polyps, enlarged tonsils
MSK	Obesity, weak muscle tone
Endocrine	Acromegaly, hypothyroidism
Medications	Alcohol, sedatives, depressants, muscle relaxants
Neurological	Stroke, myasthenia gravis

Approach to Management

Snoring is often a sign of disrupted airflow during sleep and can range from a benign condition to an indicator of more serious health concerns. A thorough history, physical examination, targeted investigations, and lifestyle or medical management approaches can help manage symptoms effectively and reduce associated health risks [19]. On examination assess the patient's nasal passages, tonsils, and uvula for obstructions or abnormalities.

Blood tests	FBC, U&E's, TFT's
	Glucose, HbA1c
	Arterial blood gases
	Plasma metanephrines (consider pseudophaeochromocytoma)
Other	Overnight sleep pulse oximetry
	Polysomnography
Imaging	Nasal endoscopy
Treatment	Lifestyle and behavioural changes
	Weight loss
	Sleep positioning
	Smoking cessation
	CPAP
	Treat the underlying cause
Red flags	Elevated ESS score, daytime somnolence and apnoeas
	Morning headaches
	Polycythaemia

SORE THROAT = pain, scratchiness or irritation in the throat, a very common presenting complaint. Also referred to as pharyngitis [20]

Characterisation
- How would you describe the pain?
- Is it scratchy, burning, sharp or raw?
- Whereabouts is the pain?
- Is the pain localised or spreading to other areas such as your ears?
- Within the mouth itself, back of the throat, lower down, all over?
- Is there radiation to the neck, ears or elsewhere?
- How intense is the pain on a scale of 1 to 10?

The throat is a very sensitive region and severe pain can be extremely problematic.

Onset + Duration
- When did it start / how long has it been going on for?
- Is it constant or intermittent?

Clarify the timeframe and check if it is present all of the time. Acute vs. chronic.

Swallowing
- Does the pain change with swallowing?

Odynophagia is a concerning sign. Find out if the pain occurs early or late and whether food is getting stuck.

- Are you having any problems with swallowing itself?

Dysphagia question set below.

Associated Symptoms
- Do you have a cough, nasal congestion, or runny nose?

Suggest a coryzal illness.

- Any fever, chills, or night sweats?
- Any hoarseness or difficulty speaking?

Can be due to generalised inflammation, swelling or irritation of the larynx, misuse or overuse of the voice but also other conditions such as GORD and smoking.

- Any hearing problems?
- Ask about vertigo, hearing loss and tinnitus.
- Any change in your sense of smell?

Consider anosmia if present.

Triggers
- What worsens the pain? For example, talking, swallowing, cold air.
- Have any treatments helped?

Has the patient tried any over-the-counter medications, warm fluids, gargling with aspirin etc.

- Have you had any recent contact with anyone with a sore throat or respiratory illness?

Close contacts are a common source of upper respiratory tract infections.

- Any travel history or exposure to environmental pollutants?

Where have they been and what have they been doing?

- Have you been smoking, vaping, or had exposure to second-hand smoke?

Smoking is highly irritant.

- Do you suffer with indigestion or acid reflux?

Common indirect cause of sore throats.

Common Causes of Sore Throat [21]

Infections	**Viral:** common cold, influenza, infectious mononucleosis, COVID-19, coxsackievirus.
	Bacterial: group A streptococcus (streptococcal pharyngitis), diphtheria, gonococcal pharyngitis.
	Fungal: Candida infections, often seen in immunocompromised individuals.
ENT	Sinusitis / postnasal drip irritating the throat.
	Tonsillitis, peritonsillar abscess, epiglottitis.
GI	Gastroesophageal reflux disease (GORD).
Immune	Allergic rhinitis, SLE / Sjogren's (cause dry mouth and throat discomfort)
Environmental	Toxins, pollutants, vaping, smoking, chemical inhalation, dry air.

Approach to Management

ENT examination is important to assess the extent of irritation and to visualise any potential airway compromise [21, 22].

Blood tests	FBC, U&E's
	Inflammatory markers
Other	Throat swab culture
	Rapid antigen detection test (RADT)
	EBV serology
	COVID-19 PCR / antigen test
Imaging	Laryngoscopy
	CXR (if indicated)
	Upper GI endoscopy (if indicated)
Treatment	Supportive measures
	Analgesia
	Hydration
	Saltwater / aspirin gargles
	Treat the underlying cause
Red flags	Stridor or respiratory compromise
	Drooling and inability to swallow
	Signs of sepsis

DYSPHAGIA = difficulty in swallowing [23]

Onset + Duration
• When did it start / how long has it been going on for?

Progressive worsening over weeks to months suggests an oesophageal malignancy.
An oesophageal ring can present intermittently.
Globus can be present for a prolonged period of time but with no other systemic upset.

Circumstances
• Does the difficulty in swallowing affect both solid foods as well as liquids?

If both are affected, then a motility or upper GI (pharyngeal) problem is most likely.
If the problem starts with solids and then liquids, then the development of a stricture is likely.

Odynophagia
• Is it painful to swallow?

Indicates either severe GORD, malignancy, achalasia or oesophageal spasm.

Difficulty Initiating Swallowing
• Do you get any coughing, choking or regurgitation?

Suggests an oropharyngeal lesion or a bulbar palsy.

Risk Factors
• Are you a smoker or drink much alcohol?
• Have you previously suffered with indigestion / heartburn symptoms?
• Have you lost any weight recently?

The responses provide clues to underlying malignancy.
Important to quantify any weight loss / change in dress size / loose clothing.

Common Causes of Dysphagia [23]

GI	Mechanical blockage e.g. Oesophageal cancer. Pharyngeal pouch
	Oesophagitis secondary to GORD, oesophageal strictures / webs
	Foreign bodies causing obstruction
	Motility problems due to achalasia, diffuse oesophageal spasm
	Hiatus hernia
Neurological	Stroke, Parkinson's disease, multiple sclerosis
Infections	Candida oesophagitis, HSV, CMV
Rheumatological	Systemic sclerosis, Sjogren's syndrome, SLE
Medications	Bisphosphonates, anti-cholinergics, NSAID's
Psychological	Globus / functional, anxiety

Approach to Management

Examine for any features of chronic liver disease, anaemia, malnutrition, and lymphadenopathy. Look for features of any systemic illness, weight loss, malignancy [23, 24].

Blood tests	FBC to test for anaemia
	U&E's to assess for dehydration and AKI
	Inflammatory markers
Imaging	Barium swallow or upper GI endoscopy depending on local guidelines
Treatment	Identify and treat the underlying cause, ENT review if oropharyngeal cause suspected, speech and language therapist assessment to assist with practicalities of swallowing, dietician review
Red flags	Odynophagia, constant and worsening or complete dysphagia

NECK LUMPS = the neck is an anatomically complex region and pathology of the underlying structures can present in a variety of ways [25]

Characterisation
- Where is the lump(s)?
- Is the lump fixed or movable?
- Is it soft, firm, or hard?

Location and characteristics are important as they give a clue to the structures of origin.

- Do you feel any pulsation?

A pulsatile lump is suggestive of a bruit in an overactive / enlarged thyroid.

Onset + Duration
- When did you first notice the lump?
- Has it changed in size, shape, or consistency over time?

An acute development of a lump is more consistent with infection or haemorrhage. Slow growing lumps may be more suggestive of a malignancy.

Associated Symptoms
- Have you had a sore throat or any cold / flu-like illnesses?

Could this be lymphadenopathy related to an infection (local or systemic).

- Have you noticed any recent weight loss, fevers, or night sweats?
- Any hoarseness or voice changes?
- Any difficulty swallowing or breathing?

Check for compromise of surrounding structures.

- Have you had any symptoms of thyroid dysfunction, such as weight changes, palpitations, temperature intolerance?

Thyroid dysfunction is common and both overactive and underactive thyroids can cause gland enlargement and lumps.

Triggers
- Any recent head or neck trauma?
- Any recent dental work / surgery?
- Any recent skin, respiratory or dental infections?
- Any recent radiation exposure?
  Are there problems in the neighbourhood.
- Any recent travel or exposure to tuberculosis (TB) or other infectious agents?

Ask about close contacts.

Malignancy Risk
- Personal history of cancers, particularly thyroid or skin cancer?
- Any history of cancer in the family?

Make sure you run through common cancer types and all first-degree family members.

Common Causes of Neck Lumps [26]

Infections	Lymphadenitis (secondary to bacterial or viral infections), Infectious mononucleosis, TB, HIV
Malignancy	Lymphoma, metastatic carcinoma, thyroid cancer, ENT tumours
Congenital	Thyroglossal duct cyst, branchial cleft cyst, dermoid cyst
Endocrine	Thyroid nodules, goitre, parathyroid adenoma (rare)
Vascular	Carotid body tumour

Approach to Management

When evaluating a patient with a neck lump, it's essential to take a comprehensive history, detailed examination, consider differential diagnoses based on the patient's age, presentation, and systemic causes, conduct appropriate investigations, and provide optimal management [27].

Blood tests	FBC, U&E's, LFT's, TFT's
	Inflammatory markers
Imaging	Neck ultrasound +/− fine needle aspiration biopsy
	CT / MRI scan
Other	Excisional biopsy
	Spirometry if airway compromise
	Upper GI endoscopy or Ba swallow if swallowing problems
Treatment	Supportive treatment
	Treat the underlying cause
Red flags	Fixed, hard lump
	Associated systemic symptoms
	Dysphagia or hoarseness
	Cardiovascular compromise relating to thyroid disease
	Painless, persistent lymph node enlargement

INTERESTING FACT: Humans can distinguish over 10,000 different scents. In fact, the nose has close to 400 types of scent receptors that can detect about 1 trillion distinct smells [28].

References

1. Hayois L, Dunsmore A. Common and serious ENT presentations in primary care. InnovAiT. 2023;16(2):79–86.
2. Emerick KS, Deschler DG. Common ENT disorders. South Med J. 2006;99(10):1090–9.
3. Gilani S. Seven cardinal questions for the patient with ear, nose or throat complaints. Review Medicine (Baltimore). 2022;16;101(50):e31852.
4. Earwood JS, Rogers TS, Rathjen NA. Ear pain: diagnosing common and uncommon causes. Am Fam Physician. 2018;97(1):20–7.
5. Hwa TP. Brant, JA. (2021) evaluation and management of otalgia. Med Clin North Am. 2021;105(5):813–26.
6. Fishman JM, Cullen L. Investigating sudden hearing loss in adults. BMJ. 2018;363(k4347)
7. Michels TC, Duffy MT, Rogers DJ. Hearing loss in adults: differential diagnosis and treatment. Am Fam Physician. 2019;100(2):98–108.
8. NICE. Hearing loss in adults: assessment and management. National Institute for Health and Care Excellence; 2023. http://www.nice.org.uk
9. BMJ Best Practice (2024) Overview of Vertigo. https://bestpractice.bmj.com/topics/en-gb/965
10. Post RE, Dickerson LM. Dizziness: a diagnostic approach. Am Fam Physician. 2010;82(4):361–8. 369
11. Dommaraju S, Perera E. An approach to vertigo in general practice. Aust Fam Physician. 2016;45:4.
12. Knight A. The differential diagnosis of rhinorrhea. J Allergy Clin Immunol. 1995;95(5):1080–3.
13. Abuzeid MO. Nasal obstruction and rhinorrhea. In: Elzouki AY, Harfi HA, Nazer HM, Stapleton FB, Oh W, Whitley RJ, editors. Textbook of clinical pediatrics. Berlin: Springer; 2012.
14. Piccirillo JF, Merritt MG Jr, Richards ML. Psychometric and clinimetric validity of the 20-item Sino-nasal outcome test (SNOT-20). Otolaryngol Head Neck Surg. 2002;126(1):41–7. https://doi.org/10.1067/mhn.2002.121022. PMID: 11821764
15. Boesveldt S, Postma EM, Boak D, Welge-Luessen A, Schöpf V, Mainland JD, Martens J, Ngai J, Duffy VB. Anosmia-A Clinical Review. Chem Senses. 2017;42(7):513–23.
16. Deutsch P, Evans C, Wahid N, Amlani A, Khanna A. Anosmia: an evidence-based approach to diagnosis and management in primary care. Br J Gen Pract. 2021;71(704):135–8.
17. Kim SG, Cho SW, Kim JW. Definition of the snoring episode index based on the analyses of snoring parameters and the apnea hypopnea index. Sci Rep. 2022;12:6761.
18. Dzieciolowska-Baran E, Gawlikowska-Sroka A, Czerwinski F. Snoring—the role of the laryngologist in diagnosing and treating its causes. Eur J Med Res. 2009;4(Suppl 4):67–70.
19. Al-Hussaini A, Berry S. An evidence-based approach to the management of snoring in adults. Clin Otolaryngol. 2015;40(2):79–85.
20. Vincent MT, Celestin N, Hussain AN. Pharyngitis. Am Fam Physician. 2004;15;69(6):1465–70.
21. Gunnarsson RK, Ebell M, Centor R, Little P, Verheij T, Lindbæk M, Sundvall PD. Best management of patients with an acute sore throat—a critical analysis of current evidence and a consensus of experts from different countries and traditions. Infect Dis. 2023;55(6):384–95.
22. BMJ Best Practice (2024) Acute pharyngitis. https://bestpractice.bmj.com/topics/en-gb/5
23. Wilkinson JM, Codipilly DC, Wilfahrt RP. Dysphagia: evaluation and collaborative management. Am Fam Physician. 2021;103(2):97–106. PMID: 33448766
24. Ahmed I, Matull R. Swallowing difficulties (dysphagia). In: Haydock S, Whitehead D, Fritz Z, editors. Acute medicine: a symptom-based approach. Cambridge University Press; 2014. p. 421–7.
25. Haynes J, Arnold KR, Aguirre-Oskins C, Chandra S. Evaluation of neck masses in adults. Am Fam Physician. 2015;91(10):698–706.

26. Bailey S, Wallwork B. Differentiating between benign and malignant thyroid nodules: an evidence-based approach in general practice. Aust J Gen Pract. 2018;47(11):770–4.
27. Pynnonen MA, Gillespie MB, Roman B, et al. Clinical practice guideline: evaluation of the neck mass in adults. Otolaryngol Head Neck Surg. 2017;157(S2):1–30.
28. Bushdid C, Magnasco MO, Vosshall LB, Keller A. Humans can discriminate more than 1 trillion olfactory stimuli. Science. 2014;21;343(6177):1370–2.

Chapter 14
Psychiatry

Abstract Mental health disorders and our awareness of them are significantly on the rise. Society and clinical medicine still struggle to be sensitive and understanding towards psychiatric issues and unfortunately there is still stigma attached. Being patient and empathetic towards individuals is key to taking a psychiatric history. Many thoughts and feelings can be difficult to articulate, and history is rife with psychiatric misdiagnoses of medical conditions and vice versa. A move away from the era of paternalistic and dismissive attitudes is essential to supporting patients the best that we can.

Keywords Psychiatry · Psychology · Mental health · Depression · Anxiety · Suicide · Thought disorder · Psychosis · Bipolar · Schizophrenia

Introduction

Effective medical history taking is the cornerstone of psychiatric assessment, providing a comprehensive understanding of a patient's mental health and overall wellbeing. Unlike other medical specialties, psychiatry places particular emphasis on exploring the biopsychosocial dimensions of a patient's life, encompassing family, environmental, psychological, and social factors. By knowing what to ask and why and mastering the art and science of psychiatric history taking, clinicians can create a foundation for compassionate, patient-centred care and advance the practice of mental health treatment [1]. Table 14.1 lists common presenting problems that are related to psychological and psychiatric conditions. Table 14.2 lists common disorders and associated symptoms.

P. Grant, *The Concise Guide to Medical History Taking*, https://doi.org/10.1007/978-3-031-91474-4_14

Table 14.1 Summary table of psychiatric presenting complaints and differential diagnoses [2]

Presenting complaints in Psychiatry	Commonly associated conditions
Low mood	Depression, bipolar disorders, bereavement, hypothyroidism, medication side effects
Stress / anxiety / panic	Anxiety disorders, GAD, social phobias, panic disorders, PTSD, hyperthyroidism, substance use and abuse / withdrawal
Mania	Bipolar disorder, substance use and abuse, thyrotoxicosis, medication side effects e.g. steroids
Delusions and hallucinations	Schizophrenia, schizoaffective disorder, bipolar disorder, delirium, dementia, substance use and abuse
Self-harm / suicidal ideation	Major depression, bipolar disorder, personality disorders, anxiety disorders, substance abuse, PTSD
Obsessions and compulsions	OCD, body dysmorphic disorders, anxiety disorders, Tourette's syndrome
Confusion / disorientation	Delirium, dementia, trauma, substance use and abuse, vitamin B12 and thiamine deficiencies
Paranoia	Schizophrenia spectrum disorders, delusional disorders, substance use and abuse, personality disorders, dementia
Impulsivity	ADHD, bipolar disorder, or personality disorders, substance use and abuse, frontal lobe injuries
Psychomotor agitation	Anxiety, mania, bipolar disorder, depression with agitation. Medication side effects e.g. Stimulants, SSRI'S. Alcohol withdrawal
Psychomotor retardation	Major depressive disorder, catatonia, dementia, Parkinson's disease, medication side effects e.g. anti-psychotics, sedatives
Sexual dysfunction	Depression, anxiety, medication side effects e.g. anti-depressants, beta blockers. Hypogonadism, menopause, substance use and abuse
Eating related complaints	Anorexia nervosa, bulimia nervosa, binge eating disorder, depression, thyroid dysfunction
Somatic complaints	Somatic symptom disorder / functional complaints, GAD, panic disorder, depression, chronic pain conditions

Table 14.2 Summary table of common Psychiatric conditions and associated symptoms [3]

Common psychiatric conditions	Common symptoms
Depression	Persistent low mood, sadness, or emptiness Loss of interest or pleasure in activities (anhedonia) Fatigue or low energy Changes in appetite or weight (increase or decrease) Sleep disturbances (insomnia or hypersomnia) Feelings of worthlessness or excessive guilt Difficulty concentrating or making decisions Physical symptoms (e.g., aches, headaches) without clear cause
Anxiety	Excessive, uncontrollable worry about various aspects of life Restlessness or feeling "on edge" Muscle tension Fatigue due to mental and physical tension Difficulty concentrating or "mind going blank" Irritability Sleep disturbances (trouble falling or staying asleep) Physical symptoms (e.g. palpitations, sweating, nausea)

(continued)

Table 14.2 (continued)

Common psychiatric conditions	Common symptoms
Bipolar disorder	**Manic symptoms:** Elevated or irritable mood Increased energy and activity levels Reduced need for sleep Rapid speech or racing thoughts Impulsivity or engaging in risky behaviours Increased self-esteem or grandiosity **Depressive symptoms** (similar to depression above) **Hypomanic symptoms** (less severe than mania but similar in presentation)
Post-traumatic stress disorder (PTSD)	Intrusive memories, flashbacks, or nightmares related to the traumatic event Avoidance of places, people, or thoughts associated with the trauma Negative changes in mood and cognition (e.g. feelings of detachment, negative beliefs) Hyperarousal symptoms (e.g. hypervigilance, exaggerated startle response) Difficulty sleeping or concentrating Irritability or angry outbursts
Schizophrenia	**Positive symptoms:** Hallucinations (often auditory) Delusions (fixed false beliefs) Disorganised speech or thought patterns Disorganised or catatonic behaviour **Negative symptoms:** Flat affect (reduced emotional expression) Poverty of speech Anhedonia (lack of pleasure) Social withdrawal or reduced motivation Cognitive symptoms, such as difficulty with memory, attention, or executive function
Psychosis	**Hallucinations** - sensory experiences without external stimuli (e.g. hearing voices) **Delusions** - strong beliefs that are contrary to reality (e.g. Paranoid or grandiose beliefs) **Disorganised thinking** - difficulty organising thoughts, leading to incoherent speech **Disorganised or abnormal behaviour** - unpredictable or inappropriate behaviour **Negative symptoms** - flat affect, reduced speaking, social withdrawal (similar to schizophrenia)
Obsessive compulsive disorder (OCD)	**Obsessions** - intrusive, repetitive thoughts, urges, or images causing anxiety (e.g. fear of contamination, harm) **Compulsions** - repetitive behaviours or mental acts performed to reduce anxiety (e.g. washing, checking, counting) Awareness that obsessions and compulsions are excessive but unable to control them. Time-consuming activities interfering with daily life and causing distress.
Personality disorders	**Cluster A (odd/eccentric):** Paranoid personality disorder - distrust and suspicion of others. Schizoid personality disorder - detachment from social relationships, limited emotion. Schizotypal personality disorder - odd beliefs, eccentric behaviour, social anxiety. **Cluster B (dramatic/emotional):** Borderline personality disorder (BPD) - intense emotions, fear of abandonment, impulsive behaviours. Narcissistic personality disorder - grandiosity, need for admiration, lack of empathy. Histrionic personality disorder - excessive emotionality, attention-seeking behaviour. Antisocial personality disorder: Disregard for others' rights, lack of remorse, impulsivity. **Cluster C (anxious/fearful):** Avoidant personality disorder - fear of rejection, feelings of inadequacy, social inhibition. Dependent personality disorder - need to be cared for, difficulty making decisions independently. Obsessive-compulsive personality disorder (OCPD) - preoccupation with orderliness, perfectionism, and control.

(continued)

Table 14.2 (continued)

Common psychiatric conditions	Common symptoms
Eating disorders	**Anorexia nervosa**: Intense fear of gaining weight or becoming "fat" Restriction of food intake leading to significantly low body weight. Distorted body image or self-worth based on weight and shape **Bulimia nervosa**: Episodes of binge eating with a lack of control Compensatory behaviours (e.g. vomiting, excessive exercise, laxative use) Self-worth tied to body shape and weight **Binge eating disorder**: Recurrent episodes of binge eating without compensatory behaviours Eating large quantities of food in a short period, feeling guilty or embarrassed afterwards

Background History in Psychiatry

Past medical and psychiatric history as well as understanding the family history, social set up and context that your patient is experiencing can be extremely useful when it comes to ascertaining a diagnosis [4]. Signal to the patient that you will be covering many areas of their life in order to build a full picture.

- History of previous medical or psychiatric problems? When were they diagnosed and by whom? What treatments did you receive?
- Have you ever been on any medication for a mental health issue?
- Have you ever received any counselling or talking therapies? Did this help?
- Are you currently under the care of mental health services? Do you have a CPN (community psychiatric nurse) or support worker?
- Have you ever been admitted to Hospital before because of a mental health issue?
- Do they have a family history of any mental health problems?
- Medications—multiple drugs, both prescribed and recreational, as well as alcohol can affect psychological well-being. Make sure that you get a full list of what they are taking.
- Constitutional upset—have you lost any weight recently? Have your diet or eating patterns changed? Don't forget to undertake a systems review in order to assess for potential underlying medical problems e.g. thyroid disorders, phaeochromocytoma, space occupying lesions etc.

LOW MOOD = feelings of sadness, unhappiness, lack of enjoyment, which may progress to deeper feelings of hopelessness, helplessness and worthlessness [5]

Characterisation
- Can you describe how you are feeling?
- Ask them to articulate their feelings in their own words.

Are they down, depressed or hopeless?

- Over the past 2 weeks have you lost interest or pleasure in doing things?

Try to establish the frequency of these feelings.

Onset + Duration
- When did you start feeling this way?
- How long has it been going on for?
- Does your mood fluctuate, or is it constant?

Duration and time course are important.

Precipitants
- Were there any significant life events or stressors before these feelings started?
Is there an identifiable trigger.

- Do you use alcohol, recreational drugs, or prescription medications that may impact your mood?

Multiple substances can cause deterioration of mood.

Impact
- Has low mood affected your ability to work, study, or engage in daily activities?
Has the individual begun to withdraw from their normal functioning.

- Do you feel fatigued?
- How is your energy throughout the day?

Tiredness and exhaustion are common features of depression.

- Have you noticed changes in your appetite or weight?

Anorexia or hyperphagia are both influenced by low mood.

- How is your sleep?
- Do you experience insomnia, early waking, or excessive sleeping?

Sleep disturbance is frequently reported in depression which exacerbates feelings of low mood.

- Do you have trouble focusing or remembering things?
- Poor concentration and memory?
- Have you noticed any changes in your sex drive?

Ask about loss of libido.

- Do you have any thoughts of self-harm or suicide?
- Have you made any previous attempts?

Ask this in a gentle and sympathetic way. Important to assess risk.

Common Causes of Low Mood [6]

Psychological	Depression, bipolar disorder, adjustment disorder, PTSD
Neurological	Dementia, Parkinson's disease, multiple sclerosis, stroke, TBI
Endocrine	Hypothyroidism, diabetes mellitus, hypogonadism, menopause
Iatrogenic	Beta blockers, steroids, anti-hypertensives
Lifestyle	Alcohol and substance abuse, poor diet, vitamin deficiencies, sleep deprivation

Approach to Management

Assessing low mood requires a thorough and sensitive approach, along with targeted investigations [7]. There are multiple psychological, psychiatric and medical causes for low mood.

Blood tests	FBC, U&E's, LFT's, TFT's
	Vitamin B12 and folate levels
	Inflammatory markers
Imaging	CT / MRI brain (if indicated)
Treatment	Identify and remove the triggers where possible
	Diet and lifestyle modifications
	Social support
	Talking therapies
	Psychoeducation
	Relaxation techniques, mindfulness etc.
	Anti-depressant medication
Red flags	Suicidal ideation
	Thought disorders
	Severe functional impairment
	Substance withdrawal

ANXIETY = a feeling of stress, worry, agitation, being on-edge, inner turmoil [8]

Characterisation
- How would you describe the way that you've been feeling?
- Have you been worrying a lot about things recently?

Individuals can explain anxiety related feelings in a variety of ways and it may often manifest in physical symptoms.

Onset + Duration
- When did you start feeling anxious?
- How long has it been going on for?

Time course and relation to life events can be very telling.

- How long do the feelings last?
- How often do you feel this way?

Is this intermittent, free-floating or continuous.

Triggers
- Was there any specific event or precipitant?
- Have you been able to identify any specific situations, people, or environments that trigger your anxiety?

Anxiety may be very situation specific or generalised with no identifiable trigger.

- Are you able to put your worries out of your mind or control your anxiety?

It's useful to know if they have developed coping strategies or distraction techniques.

- Are you on any medications?
- Do you consume alcohol, nicotine, caffeine, or recreational drugs?

Are they taking any stimulants or narcotics that may be interfering?

Impact
- How is this affecting your life?
- Do you avoid doing things, people, places because of your worries?

What is the impact on the individual's life and day to day activities. They may no longer be able to work or leave the house.

- Do you get sudden 'attacks' of anxiety or panic?

Exacerbations of anxiety and panic attacks can be very distressing.

Associated Symptoms
- Do you experience palpitations, shortness of breath, sweating, muscle tension, nausea, or headaches?

Physical symptoms of anxiety can be very uncomfortable.

- Has your anxiety affected your sleep patterns e.g. difficulty falling or staying asleep, nightmares?

Sleep disturbance is very common with anxiety and can perpetuate the problem.

- Has your appetite changed?
- More or less?
- Do you have difficulty concentrating or feel distracted?

The racing mind may make it difficult to focus and function.

- Have you ever felt detached from yourself or your surroundings?

Consider depersonalisation and derealisation.

Common Causes of Anxiety [9]

Psychological	**Primary Anxiety Disorders:** Generalised Anxiety Disorder (GAD), Panic Disorder, Social Anxiety Disorder, Specific Phobias, and Obsessive-Compulsive Disorder (OCD)
	Anxiety co-existent with depression
	Post-traumatic stress disorder
Neurological	Temporal lobe epilepsy, Parkinson's disease
Endocrine	Hyperthyroidism, hypoglycaemia, Phaeochromocytoma (rare)
Lifestyle	Stimulants such as caffeine, nicotine, amphetamines
	Alcohol and drug withdrawal

Approach to Management

Addressing anxiety with a patient, structured approach can help identify the underlying cause, provide appropriate management, and recognise when urgent intervention is necessary [10].

Blood tests	FBC, U&E's, TFT's
	Inflammatory markers
	Random glucose levels
	Plasma metanephrines (if indicated)
Other	ECG
	Urine toxicology
Treatment	Identify and alleviate the underlying cause
	Lifestyle management, exercise, sleep hygiene
	Psychoeducation
	Psychotherapy / counselling / talking therapies
	Medications (if indicated)
Red flags	Rapidly escalating symptoms (may indicate a medical issue)
	Severe suicidal ideation
	Thought disorder
	Autonomic instability / cardiovascular compromise

THOUGHT DISORDERS = a disorganised way of thinking. This is a mental health condition that affects a person's ability to think clearly and logically. It can impact a person's ability to communicate, interpret reality, and perform daily tasks [11]

Characterisation
- Do you think that the way that you've been thinking has changed?

What is their take on the way that they have been thinking and feeling. It's useful to get a verbatim quote 'like angels are forcing me to think this way'.

- In what way would you describe this?
- Do you feel that others find it difficult to understand you or follow your train of thought?
- Have you had any strange or intrusive thoughts, or felt that your mind is racing or slowing down?

Onset + Duration
- How long have you noticed unusual or disorganised thoughts for?

Has this always been a part of their lives or gradually developed recently. When did it become apparent to them that they had a problem.

Triggers
- Have you had any recent head injuries, seizures, or memory loss?
- Have you experienced any recent major life events or stress?

Rule out a traumatic brain injury, situational stressors, post-ictal phenomena or other neuro-degenerative conditions.

Impact
- How has this affected your daily functioning, work, or relationships?
- Are you able to concentrate or focus as usual?

What is the impact on their life and those around them.

Perception
- Do you feel confused about what is real versus what is imagined?
- Have you experienced any unusual beliefs or suspicions about others?
- Can anyone hear your thoughts?

Clarify if they are they struggling to work out what is real, or becoming paranoid.

- Do you ever hear noises or voices when there is nobody else there?
- Are the voices talking about you or talking to you?

Suggestive of auditory hallucinations

- Do you sometimes have thoughts that others tell you are false?
- Do you have any beliefs that aren't shared by others you know?

Suggestive of delusional thinking

- Is there anyone taking thoughts out of your head or putting thoughts in?

Thought withdrawal / insertion.

- Do you ever hear your own thoughts echoed or repeated?

Thought echo.

Associated Symptoms
- Do you feel unusually anxious, fearful, or suspicious of others?
- Have you had changes in mood, energy, or motivation?
- Any recent sleep disturbances or changes in appetite?

Alongside the thought disorder clarify what other mental health or physical problems they may be experiencing.

Common Causes of Thought Disorders [12]

Psychiatric	**Schizophrenia Spectrum Disorders** - often associated with thought disorganisation, illogical thinking, and hallucinations
	Mood disorders - severe depression or bipolar disorder may present with impaired thought patterns, such as depressive rumination or manic racing thoughts
	Obsessive-compulsive disorder (OCD) - intrusive thoughts and obsessive preoccupations can appear disorganised to an observer
Neurological	Dementia and cognitive disorders e.g. Alzheimer's or Lewy body
	Delirium - acute confusional state
	Traumatic brain injury
	Post-ictal
Substances	Alcohol, cannabis, stimulants, hallucinogens, opiates.
	Withdrawal states especially alcohol and benzodiazpenes.
Metabolic	Hypothyroidism can lead to impaired cognition, hyperthyroidism can cause agitation and thought disturbance.
	Hyponatraemia, hypercalcaemia
Infections	CNS infections such as meningitis and encephalitis
	Systemic sepsis, especially in the elderly e.g. UTI'S

Approach to Management

Thought disorder requires a thorough approach to understanding its origin and determining the appropriate intervention. Management focuses on treating the underlying condition, whether psychiatric, neurological, or medical, while prioritising patient safety and providing support for long-term recovery [13].

Blood tests	FBC, U&E's, LFT's, B12 & Folate
	Calcium studies
	Inflammatory markers
	Blood glucose
Other	EEG (if seizure activity suspected)
	Neuropsychological testing
Imaging	CT / MRI brain
Treatment	Supportive measures
	Treat the underlying cause
	Medications appropriate to the condition
	Psychotherapy / psychoeducation
Red flags	Severe psychosis symptoms
	Suicidal ideation or self harm
	Sudden onset of symptoms
	Focal neurological signs

CONFUSION = cognitive impairment, change in mental state, memory problems, ability to think, use judgement and make decisions. Collateral history is very helpful [14]

Characterisation
- Can you describe what problems you've been having with your thinking and memory recently?

Start with a general description of what they have been experiencing before you get into any specifics.

- Are you experiencing any of the following; agitation, aggression, hallucinations, delusions, wandering?

Features of hyperactive delirium.

- Or alternatively any of; sleepiness, lethargy, slowing down, poor attention?

Features of hypoactive delirium.

Onset + Duration
- When did it start / how long has it been going on for?
- Has it been intermittent, worsening, or stable?

A collateral history may be most useful here to get an objective assessment.
Is this an acute state (delirium) or chronic (dementia).

- Is the confusion constant or does it fluctuate?

Clarify if the confusion is worse at certain times of the day.

Precipitants
- Have there been any recent problems with your health? For example, infections, trauma, dehydration, medication changes e.g. sedatives, opioids, anticholinergics?
- Any accompanying fever, headache, vision changes, seizures, or weakness?
- Any recent falls or head injuries?

Sub-dural haematomas can slowly increase pressure on the brain and present with confusion.

- Any changes in alcohol intake or drug use recently?

Consider intoxication or withdrawal.

- Any changes in your home / living environment or any major life events?

Situational changes can be disorientating for susceptible individuals.

Memory
- Are there problems with short-term or long-term memory?

Asking specifically about each of these aspects of cognitive performance helps to narrow down the potential structures and systems that are affected and are a useful measure of global performance.

Concentration
- Do you have difficulty focusing on tasks or conversations?

Communication
- Do you have any problems with speaking or understanding?

Decision-making
- Have you had any problems with making decisions or poor judgement?

Orientation
- Do you know whereabouts you are right now?
- Do you who know who I am?
- Do you know what time it is?

Assess whether they are oriented to time, place and person.

Abbreviated Mental Test (AMT-10)

Allocate 1 point for a correct answer, 0 for an incorrect answer.

1. What is your age?
2. What is the time (to the nearest hour)?

I'm going to ask you to remember an address and then ask you about it later.
  Can you remember the following '42 West Street'?

3. What is the current year?
4. What is you home address?
5. What is my job? What is this object? (show the patient a simple object)
6. What is your date of birth?
7. What year did the first world war start?
8. Who is the current Prime Minister (or equivalent)?
9. Please can you count backwards down from 20 to 1?
10. Can you recall the address I asked you to remember?

This is a screening tool only [15]. A total score of 10 is normal / no confusion.
  A score < 7 suggests that cognitive impairment may be present.
  4–6 moderate impairment.
  < 3 severe cognitive impairment.

Common Causes of Confusion / Cognitive Impairment [16]

Neurological	Cerebrovascular disease, Dementia (Alzheimer's, Lewy-body, Fronto-temporal), Traumatic brain injury
	Post-ictal
	Space-occupying lesions
Infections	Systemic infections, sepsis, UTI'S.
	CNS infections; meningitis, encephalitis.
Metabolic	Hypo / hyper - glycaemia,
	Electrolyte imbalances e.g. hypercalcaemia, hyponatraemia, thyroid disorders, liver failure, renal failure (uraemia), vitamin B12 and / or thiamine deficiency.
Cardiovascular	Hypoxia, reduced cerebral perfusion, hypertensive encephalopathy, vasculitides.
Psychiatric	Psychosis, depression, anxiety, mania, sleep deprivation.
Medication	Drug intoxication, alcohol excess / withdrawal, heavy metals, CO

Approach to Management

Confusion is a non-specific symptom that can be caused by a wide variety of conditions affecting the brain and other systems. A stepwise screening approach to investigations is necessary to rule out the possible causes [17]. Immediate attention to red flags and urgent management of life-threatening conditions is critical for preventing irreversible damage.

Blood tests	FBC, U&E's, LFT's, TFT's, Calcium
	Haematinics
	Blood glucose
	Inflammatory markers
	Toxicology screen
	Arterial blood gas
Other	Urinalysis
	Lumbar puncture (if indicated)
	EEG (if seizures suspected)
Imaging	CT / MRI brain scan
	CXR
Treatment	Supportive management
	Reduce potential precipitants / environmental stimuli
	Treat the underlying cause
Red flags	Sudden onset
	Focal neurological deficits
	Meningism
	Reduced level of consciousness
	New onset seizures

SOMATIC / FUNCTIONAL SYMPTOMS = refers to the manifestations of physical symptoms that cannot be fully explained by any known medical condition - they are often related to underlying psychological factors [18]

Characterisation
- Can you describe your symptoms in detail?

Try to nail down the specifics of what the individual has been experiencing.

- Have you previously undergone tests or treatments for these symptoms, and what were the outcomes?

The individual may have a long history of medically unexplained symptoms and been to see clinicians in multiple different medical specialities searching for an explanation.

Onset + Duration
- When did it start / how long has it been going on for?
- Are the symptoms constant or intermittent?

Chart the time course and the interaction with life events and fluctuations in symptoms.

Triggers
- Are there any particular times or situations that worsen or relieve them?
- Have there been any recent stressors, life changes, or events that may correlate with the onset of symptoms?

Is there a reliable predictor of what may cause an exacerbation of the symptoms.

- Do you use any alcohol, tobacco, or recreational drugs?

Also record any herbal supplements or over the counter preparations.

Relieving Factors
- How do you cope with the symptoms?
- Do you have support from friends, family, or therapists?

What are the patient's coping strategies and support mechanisms.

Associated Symptoms
- Do you experience fatigue, sleep disturbances, or lifestyle changes (diet, exercise)?

What has the impact been of these symptoms on the individual and those around them.

- Do you suffer with irritable bowels, gastric reflux or the sensation of their being something stuck in your throat.

The GI tract frequently manifests psychological disturbances.

- Do you experience any chest pain or palpitations?

Cardiovascular symptoms are a feature of autonomic activation and stress.

- Do you hyperventilate, struggle to breathe or getting pins and needles in your fingers?

Rapid, shallow, over breathing can exacerbate symptoms and make the individual feel lightheaded or tingly due to low carbon dioxide.

- Do you experience chronic muscle aches and pains?
- Is the pain in the joints or between the joints?

Fibromyalgia often presents with a feeling of exhaustion and muscle pain.

Common Causes of Somatic / Functional Symptoms [19]

Neurological	Fibromyalgia, tension-type headaches, non-epileptic seizures, chronic fatigue syndrome / ME
Psychiatric	Anxiety, depression, panic disorder, health anxiety
Infections	Infectious conditions and post-viral syndromes can lead to a variety of non-specific signs and symptoms e.g. Lyme disease
Metabolic	Addison's disease, hypoglycaemia, dumping syndrome, vitamin D deficiency

Approach to Management

We don't know enough about functional disorders. This makes the evaluation complex, requiring a thorough empathetic history taking, investigation, and consideration of psychological and social factors. The worry is that something serious and medical may be missed or that the patient's problems are written off as being 'all in their mind' thereby doing them a great disservice [20].

Blood tests	FBC, U&E's, LFT's, TFT's, B12 and Folate
	Inflammatory markers
	Glucose monitoring
	9 AM cortisol
	Vitamin D
	Lyme serology (if indicated)
Imaging	Only if indicated

(continued)

Treatment	Identify and treat the underlying cause where possible
	Reassurance
	Diet and lifestyle
	PRN analgesia
	Regular exercise
	Mindfulness and relaxation techniques
	Social networks and support groups
	Referral to a psychiatrist or psychologist for conditions like health anxiety or somatic symptom disorder, particularly if there is significant distress or functional impairment.
Red flags	Focal neurological deficits
	Self-harm or suicidal ideation

INTERESTING FACT: Psychiatry only became a distinct medical specialty in the late 19th and early 20th centuries. The words "lunacy" and "lunatic" come from the Roman goddess of the moon, Luna, and the belief that the moon influenced mental health and behaviour, such as the increases in A&E attendances during periods of the full moon [21].

References

1. Stein DJ, Shoptaw SJ, Vigo DV, Lund C, Cuijpers P, Bantjes J, Sartorius N, Maj M. Psychiatric diagnosis and treatment in the 21st century: paradigm shifts versus incremental integration. World Psychiatry. 2022 Oct;21(3):393–414.
2. NICE. Common mental health problems: identification and pathways to care Clinical guideline [CG123]. 2011. https://www.nice.org.uk/guidance/cg123
3. van Niekerk M, et al. The Prevalence of Psychiatric Disorders in General Hospital Inpatients: A Systematic Umbrella Review. J Acad Consult-Liaison Psychiatry. 2022;63(6):567–78. ISSN 2667-2960
4. Moldawsky RJ. Is the psychiatric history losing its relevance? Perm J. 2020;24:19.186.
5. NICE. When should I suspect a diagnosis of depression? Clinical Knowledge Summary. 2024. https://cks.nice.org.uk/topics/depression/diagnosis/diagnosis/
6. Kessler RC, Bromet EJ. The epidemiology of depression across cultures. Annu Rev Public Health. 2013;34:119–38.
7. Ferenchick EK, Ramanuj P, Pincus HA. Depression in primary care: part 1— screening and diagnosis. Br Med J. 2019;365:l794.
8. BMJ. Generalised anxiety disorder. In: BMJ Best Practice. BMJ Publishing Group; 2021. https://bestpractice.bmj.com/info.
9. Craske M, Stein M. Anxiety. Lancet. 2016;388:3048–59.
10. Penninx BW, Pine DS, Holmes EA, et al. Anxiety disorders. Lancet. 2021;397(10277):914–27.
11. Sass L, Parnas J. Thought disorder, subjectivity, and the self. Schizophr Bull. 2017;43(3):497–502.
12. Passby L, Broome MR. Thought disorder. BJ Psych Advances. 2017;23(5):321–3.
13. Andreasen NC. Thought disorder. In: Fatemi SH, Clayton PJ, editors. The medical basis of psychiatry. 3rd ed. Humana Press/Springer Nature; 2008. p. 435–43.
14. Roy E. Cognitive Impairment. In: Gellman MD, Turner JR, editors. Encyclopedia of behavioral medicine. New York: Springer; 2013.

15. Hodkinson HM. Evaluation of a mental test score for assessment of mental impairment in the elderly. Age Ageing. 1972;1(4):233–8.
16. Knopman DS. Cognitive impairment and other dementias. In: Goldman L, Schafer AI, editors. Goldman-Cecil medicine. 26th ed. Philadelphia, PA: Elsevier; 2020. Chap 374.
17. Galvin, J. Sadowsky, C (2012) Practical guidelines for the recognition and diagnosis of dementia. J Am Board Fam Med 25(3), 367–382.
18. Sharpe M. Somatic symptom and related disorders. In: Firth J, Conlon C, Cox T, editors. Oxford textbook of medicine. 6th ed. Oxford: Oxford University Press; 2020.
19. McGeary DD, Hartzell MM, McGeary CA, Gatchel RJ. Somatic disorders. In: Norcross JC, VandenBos GR, Freedheim DK, Pole N, editors. APA handbook of clinical psychology: psychopathology and health. American Psychological Association; 2016. p. 209–23.
20. Löwe B, et al. Persistent physical symptoms: definition, genesis, and management. Lancet. 2024;403(10444):2649–62.
21. Thompson D, Adams S. The full moon and ED patient volumes: unearthing a myth. Am J Emerg Med. 1996;14(2):161–4. ISSN 0735-6757

Correction to: The Concise Guide to Medical History Taking

Correction to:
P. Grant, *The Concise Guide to Medical History Taking*,
https://doi.org/10.1007/978-3-031-91474-4

In the original version of the book, the following belated corrections have been incorporated.

The section after 'Common Causes' has been updated to 'Approach to Management' in all the chapters.

© The Author(s), under exclusive license to Springer Nature
Switzerland AG 2026
P. Grant, *The Concise Guide to Medical History Taking*,
https://doi.org/10.1007/978-3-031-91474-4_15